A Journey of Dementia

Through

The Eyes of a Carer

A Journey of Dementia Through the Eyes of a Carer

By

Kat Toriez

Kat Toriez, an Australian author, has been writing from her heart for many years. She has shared poetry and fictional novels. This book offers a compelling and intimate look at her life as a caregiver for someone with dementia.

DEDICATION

This book is dedicated to Mac whose smile brought sunshine to my life every day

Jane said one day, "I wish I had known how hard the journey would be. I wish that I would have been aware of the changes that would confront me daily."

In this book, the author will take you on a journey with raw honesty and tenderness. From the initial shock and confusion to the daily challenges and heartache. To realise a decline in a relationship that is forced upon one is one step on the dementia path, but to live with it is the hardest lesson forced on anyone.

Mac was the happy-go-lucky man of Jane's life. He lived and breathed work ethics and delighted in life in general. For such a man to succumb to Alzheimer's was the cruellest element in their life. One, which they physically endured for ten years as they hesitantly took each step together in Mac's fight with forgetfulness.

The carer needs all the support he/she can muster up to face the day-to-day trials associated with dementia. Not only for guidance but friendship plays a huge role in this act. Jane eventually found that friendship and guidance, but it took every fibre of herself to keep on stepping on that troubled road.

This novel is a work of non-fiction and reflects the author's personal experiences. Character names, except Mac, have been changed but places and incidents are true and correct.

'To get through the hardest journey we need to take only one step at a time, but we must keep on stepping'

Chinese Proverbs

Contents

Chapter 1 – "Life is Good" 8

Chapter 2 - Discovery and Disclosure 13

Chapter 3 - Awareness and Acceptance 21

Chapter 4 - Speculation and Contemplation 29

Chapter 5 - Acceptance and Procedures 35

Chapter 6 - The Fallout 42

Chapter 7 - Decline and Assistance 50

Chapter 8 - The Middle of the Tunnel 59

Chapter 9 - Severe Cognitive Decline 67

Chapter 10 - A World to Live In, One to Be Believed 80

Chapter 11 - Severe Dementia 87

Chapter 12 - The Big Blue Room Behind That Locked Door ... 94

Chapter 13 - Life! Love! Loss! 101

Chapter 14 - Progression...Regression 114

Chapter 15 - Make believe it never happened 124

Chapter 16 - Once upon a Christmas time… 129

Chapter 17 - The Final Road 134

Chapter 18 - Bury the Memories 140

After Note 150

Chapter 1 – "Life is Good"

Jane's tears had settled, though they left tell-tale traces on her swollen eyes. Despair had been the mantle she had worn for the last few months. It's not every day that a mother buries her son. Her boy. Her only. Her gentle guiding beam of light.

Yet the weightlessness needed to be lifted. To allow the light of the future in. Something in the future to look forward to, with a happy heart. Not a heart that had been weighted down in sorrow.

Mac was turning sixty. Now that was a joyous occasion to look forward to. Something of a frivolous nature to make people smile again and forget the sadness of the previous months. Jane planned a surprise party for her man, and with the help of one of her daughters, the preparations had fallen into place with ease.

Mac and Jane had been married for fifteen odd years. A second marriage for both. A seemingly easy relationship. Their love for one another obvious to all. The guest list for the party was a combination of family and friends, and the venue was one where all frequented often.

The party was a great release of pent-up emotions. Above all of that, Mac was clueless to the whole charade and a bigger surprise could not have given more joy. It was wonderful to touch base with people from his past. To continue to enjoy the company of new friends and Jane had sat down with a happy heart and put that smile back on her face, ready to face the future.

Mac was a salesperson. A gifted salesman. He delighted in 'talking the talk'.

He always said, "I'm not selling anything to you, you're buying it from me."

Funny. He'd been a car salesperson most of his life. He delved into the role of management in that industry for some years and he was a respected boss, but when his age inched toward that word 'retirement' he'd moved to a different venue in the selling world and found interest in recreational vehicles.

Naturally, everyone who thought an RV was worth buying was Mac's age or more, and most of that age group, were hell bent on exploring Australia.

It was a lifestyle that he longed for as well. Mac had travelled far and wide over his home country through the years. He'd lived out west at Charleville, Queensland, for some time and he'd been a country boy at heart.

Yet the coastal beaches were appealing to him too. The laid-back lifestyle of beach goers and the fact that he'd ridden a surfboard all those years ago, as a teenager, remained a fond memory, and it seemed to be calling him back to the beach.

The beach and the ocean are elements to be consumed and enjoyed with more than a passing fancy. It offers a unique lifestyle, making a difference.

That was the enticement for he and Jane, when he wanted to get the dust out of his lungs from country living and breathe in the tangy, salty air once more. Their children were all older now. It was only the two of them to make the move to sunshine, surf and sand.

Jane did not have regular employment, though she had, over the years worked as a receptionist in offices. Then she turned her hand to sewing and being creative in a curtain shop had brought many happy days. Later, tirelessly packing biscuits at a hot and stuffy biscuit factory was not something she wanted to endure for too long.

This lifestyle at the beach was perfect. Jane felt no need to work at that present moment. One of her daughters lived on the Sunny Coast. She had two children. Grandkids for Jane and Mac to cherish and spoil.

Jane preferred to be available to mind these grand cherubs, should she be called upon to do so. Especially as their mother was furthering her studies at university and the prospect of a transfer as a teacher in the education system, loomed with good prospects.

That transfer came when Jane was not really ready to say goodbye to those little darlings or the daughter that had become more and more of a delight in their everyday life. Her move to Gladstone was some six hours car travel from the Sunny Coast.

Mac said, "It's only a hop, skip and a jump away! I'm looking forward to that drive. It will be good to see how they have settled into their new lifestyle."

Such was the life for Mac and Jane. Quiet, without the regular grandkids but other grandkids were of the age to visit in school holidays and stay and enjoy what was on offer at the beach.

That became something both looked forward to. Jane had more time to spend with the holiday makers, and Mac enjoyed the hours he could spare when possible, showing them the benefits of a coastal lifestyle.

As an RV salesperson, Mac became well known. He had secured endless accomplishments and was, at times, an Australian high-ranking seller in the recreational vehicle industry.

Jane and he had travelled when they could, or more-so, when the funds were good, to overseas countries. They enjoyed many short drive holidays in Australia when time permitted. Mac was an avid driver. He loved to be on the road. Jane delighted in his ability to make a Sunday arvo drive the perfect end to a week.

Still, he never lost 'the gift of the gab' to sell. He was a natural.

He whistled every day of his working life. He had an infectious laugh. His beautiful singing voice a given. Above all he loved his Jane. They were happy together.

Then, a niggling pain kept re-occurring in his joints. He had arthritis in one of his knees and right hip. The pain was unbearable some days. Those walks on the beach seemed at times to be a real problem and not that he was one to whinge about it, Jane knew he was struggling to walk.

Jane mused to herself wondering what to do. Obviously, try and seek out a specialist in that field. Mac had always turned his nose up at doctors. Not because he thought their job was not professional. He believed that doctors were not needed in his life. He scoffed at pain killers.

He preferred to down a beer and say, "She's right mate. All good. Tomorrow is another day."

Yep, it sure is, but Jane eventually talked him into accepting that the next day, and the next, would be oh so horrid with pain if he did nothing about it. She made an appointment for him with a GP and after much chastisement, Mac went to meet the doctor who was to become the mainstay of his life.

His famous last words that the doctor would make little money from him, was to be the irony of his life.

Chapter 2 - Discovery and Disclosure

Another great man, a specialist, came on board to give Mac a new life with new joints. It was not achieved overnight. Firstly, the hip operation. A major event in the life of someone who hardly ever darkened the door of a doctor let alone a hospital.

The usual blood tests before the op were interesting as they revealed that Mac had a B12 deficiency. This deficiency can cause a variety of symptoms including fatigue, headaches, depression and mental impairment.

Jane would never have said that Mac suffered with any of these.

Soon after the operation, whilst Mac was in four weeks of recovery, she noticed interesting signs creeping into the usual happy-go-lucky attitude of her favourite man.

He seemed pre-occupied with some of his thoughts, and he was certainly tired a lot more. Knowing that exercise with the new hip was a painstaking trial, Mac had endeavoured to make each day count and he kept up his accepted daily walk without too much indifference or reproach.

It was after the walk that an afternoon siesta ensued, and it was not only a nap; it was a good two-hour sleep.

Jane made another appointment with the GP Mac had seen before the hip operation. It was to discuss what she thought was not the 'norm' with Mac.

He was surprised to meet her on the advisory level rather than as Mac's wife. Jane explained that it was in her interest to put some of her niggling questions to the good man. He suggested a course of B12 injections. The doctor agreed that the operation certainly would have been a taxing time for his patient, especially as he had always played golf and now found it hard to even swing a club.

They had talked golf together like old pros, from the minute Mac had met him.

"I can't swing a club like I used to and my sense of direction needs repair." Mac moaned to the GP.

The doctor laughed about the situation but assured Mac that he'd be back to his good self in no time.

Within another year the arthritis in Mac's knee was hindering his usual gait. During that year, whilst Mac had returned to normal conditions at his work, he seemed to be struggling with some of the paperwork.

He was reading numbers wrongly, when he filled out a sales certificate. He laughed about it with Jane when asking for Jane's help in completing the forms. She obliged, all the while wondering if in fact, he may need an eye appointment and an upgrade in his glasses.

She never attended that eye specialist appointment with him and accepted that he had new glasses, and for once, not asking for the finer details of what had taken place at the examination.

However, Mac persisted with asking for help in writing numbers and it became another concern for Jane, for it was obvious the new glasses had made little difference.

When the two of them went once more to the surgeon who was to perform the knee replacement, Jane was hesitant. She wondered if her next request would be thought of 'unusual'.

She asked could the operation be performed with less anaesthetic, or could an alternative opiate, be used. Jane had a 'gut feeling' (and one backed up with a little research on her part) that the number of anaesthetic drugs administered throughout the hip operation may have contributed to Mac's increasing unaware state.

This operation went ahead with epidurals as a second choice. Mac sailed through his recovery and convalescence.

Mac continued with his B12 treatment. Jane felt no need to further see his GP and left Mac to make these appointments to suit his work commitments.

There was a highlight to working in the RV industry, and that was the annual rally of people and their motor homes or caravans from all over Australia. They would converge on a designated township for a reunion of old friends and a revival of past experiences and future dreams.

Mac had been an exceptional heavy vehicle licence driver for some time, and he loved to participate at these assembled nomad's events. He always achieved good sales. He would often drive an RV to the meeting place and live on site, for the duration, or in a motel close to the grounds where it was held. The whole event usually lasted one week.

He, being a recognised fun person within the RV industry, had been to previous shows, anywhere from Winton, Maryborough,

Toowoomba and Brisbane. The next big rally was to be held in Rockhampton, central Queensland, Australia.

By this time, Jane's daughter, Joanne, had settled herself and her family at Gladstone. She had slipped into the educational world like a hand in a glove.

It was decided that Jane and Mac would drive a motor home up to Gladstone. They both would stay the night with her family, and then the next morning Mac would continue to Rockhampton, roughly an hour's drive further north. Jane would stay with the daughter for those few days.

Everyone was very excited about this trip, mainly to see one another again but the highlight was to be whilst Mac was at Rockhampton, the daughter would drive the children and Jane out to see all the new caravans and RVs on display. It also gave the kids a chance to see grand-dad and get treated with an ice-cream and soft-drink.

The weather was fine and very hot in Rockhampton. The kids loved climbing up into the big home that Mac was overseeing and pretending they were in a café whilst they had their treats. There were lots of giggles and photos.

While they were all busy, Jane took the opportunity to catch up with some old friends that Mac had made over the years with his experience in selling and advising on the benefits of travelling in 'a home away from home'.

An older couple who had been wonderful friends to Mac were delighted to meet with Jane.

"Goodness. What has happened to our Macca!" was the comment they made to Jane when they had hugged and said 'hello'.

"Why do you ask?" was Jane's query.

"He's lost so much weight. He's not his usual happy self and he seems to be lost, somehow!"

"You think? Maybe the heat has got to him. It's stinking hot here today. He'd not been used to this. We get the sea breezes on the Sunny Coast." Jane replied.

"No, Jane. It's not the heat. There is something not quite right with Mac."

Jane pondered this response and, on the way back to Gladstone with her daughter, offered her thoughts to her and asked had she seen anything different with her stepfather.

Joanne responded that she could see nothing exceptionally wrong with Mac but she did add she thought he had lost weight as well.

The daughter put it down to the length of time since seeing one another. She suggested that the toll the old arthritic joints might have had on him and the subsequent operations could have contributed to his failing to look as healthy as possibly a few years earlier.

Jane and Mac always walked each day. Sometimes for Jane, more than once. Exercise had been high on the agenda for them both.

Jane was hesitant in agreeing that anything major was amiss in their lifestyle. Merely an aging process and no cause for alarm.

Mac returned after four days and having rested for another twenty-four hours with family; he and Jane resumed the trip back down to the Sunny Coast. It was not until home and Jane unpacking Mac's bag, that she found his toiletries bag missing. A belt had also been left behind. She rang her daughter and asked could she have a look for them at her place.

"Not there, I've upended everything in the room you stayed in."

Where had he left them? Jane pondered that question.

Obviously at the motel in Rockhampton. Jane rang the said place but as it had been many more hours since his stay there, with people coming and going, it was stated that nothing of that nature had been found. Mystery!

The next morning after breakfast, Mac was reading the paper seeing as it was the weekend. He bought a paper every single day. Always walking down to the newsagent and having a chat with the owners. He usually read it at work. That day was Sunday and no work.

Jane noticed something odd. Mac was wearing her reading glasses. Not her newest pair. She had two. One pair she kept in the drawer as a spare in case of emergency.

"Mac. Why have you got my glasses on?" she asked.

He looked at her vacantly. "I don't. These are mine." He replied.

Jane hesitated. "No, you have light frames. These are heavier and they have a pink tinge to them." She laughed. "Where did you get them from?" she enquired.

"In the drawer where I always keep them." He responded.

Reaching out Jane took the glasses and popped them on her face.

"They look good on you." He complimented her.

"That's because they're mine, Mac. Not yours!"

He put his head back in the chair and rested it for a while. He did not appear perturbed with the latest incident. Preferring not to offer any further words. She let it be. There was no point in stressing the obvious. Mac was oblivious to the slip-up.

Jane then went in search of his most recent spectacle prescription, wondering all the while what RV home in Rockhampton, his missing glasses could be hiding in.

The incident did not stop there. When Jane put the prescription in at her optometrist, who happened to be open and convenient at the time, she was met with a query.

"Whose script, was it?"

Naturally Jane's reply was that it belonged to her husband.

"Where and when had Mac had his eyes tested?"

Jane had to think hard, before recalling the relevant details because that was one appointment she had not attended with her husband.

Her optometrist decided to book Mac in for another appointment, even though it was obvious that he should not have been due for one. He thought something was not quite right. He was looking back over past appointments that Mac would have had, and the script Jane gave him, certainly did not make sense.

Jane had been unaware that Mac had gone to a different optometrist for a test. She had presumed that he had gone to the one which they both attended and had been attending for some years. She had not even questioned Mac's new glasses at that time. It was obvious that the script that Jane had handed over was nothing like what Mac should have been wearing. She looked worried and concerned.

"Never mind. We'll fix it all. What is your husband wearing now for reading glasses?" inquired the optometrist.

"Mine. Apparently!" Jane sheepishly acknowledged.

The man smirked and said ever so quietly. "We'll get this all sorted. He'll be good to go within the week!"

Certainly, several discoveries filtered through Jane's mind after the rally in Rockhampton. It was obvious Mac had been struggling with his eyesight. That could be the reason why he was up against a huge wall with numbers or could there be another reason.

She hoped that was not so, but at the bottom of all those thoughts one day when she was ironing Mac's trousers, she noticed they were a smaller size than what he would have worn six months previously. He had bought new work trousers for Rockhampton. She'd not checked any sizes. Mac had always bought his own work pants and his shirts were provided by the company he worked for.

She couldn't remember the last time he would have bought jeans or regular going out trousers. It was obvious that Mac had lost some weight to be wearing a smaller size. Jane went and checked the new belt that he'd bought at the markets after he lost his in Rockhampton, it was a smaller size than the other belts hanging in his wardrobe.

Then, thinking to herself, the new belt was the only one that Jane saw him wearing daily. Obviously, the others were all too big for him.

All that aside, Jane was to realise with mixed trepidation, life was becoming a little more complicated as far as Mac was concerned and not all that was happening sat easy in her mind.

Chapter 3 - Awareness and Acceptance

The outcome of the eye appointment was, to say the least, a ripple on the sand. The optometrist wondered how Mac had even been able to see with them, let alone make a difference. Within a few weeks, Mac happily donned his new reading glasses and seemed able to cope with completing his sales forms. By this time its relevance, whilst it made Jane angry, as to how it happened, all amount of questioning was a wasted time.

She was now preoccupied with plans for a little holiday over the Christmas festive season. The family were to meet at Tannum Sands Holiday Village, about a twenty-five-minute drive from Gladstone.

The get together consisted of Joanne and her crew from Gladstone and another daughter, Tia and her family from Brisbane. They were all tenting, and Mac and Jane were driving a motor home up from the Sunny Coast and camping right beside them for the week. What fun!

When Jane had travelled with Mac up to Gladstone some months previously in a motor home, for the rally in

Rockhampton, it had not entered her head that Mac could have trouble driving the huge beast.

She accepted his ever-reliable judgement and skill. She did her usual nod off after settling into the rhythm of the wheels hitting the long and winding road.

'BBBRRRPPP' 'BBBRRRPPP' Jolted awake suddenly, Jane contemplated that noise. She waited. There it was again.

She looked across at Mac driving. He seemed fine then she realised that Mac was drifting, preferring to sit on the white line on the fringe of the road. A lot more than necessary. He was not driving erratically, nor did he appear to be nodding off. He only seemed to be travelling as far left as he could.

"Hey, straighten up, can you! I don't feel like being flung into the ditch!" Jane admonished.

"What? What are you talking about. I'm sitting pretty." He chuckled.

"You're not Mac. You're driving to the left all the time. Is it the home? Is something wrong with the steering?" she asked.

"No. Look." He took his hands off the steering wheel, and it stayed steady and straight. "Maybe it could have a little something wrong, but I doubt it. It got the once over before we left the dealership."

"Well, if there is nothing wrong with it, stop driving so far over. Sit in the middle of your road."

"I am. I tell you. Stop worrying." With that once more he veered to the left. BBBRRRPPP!

"Shit Mac. Stop it. You're scaring me. This is a big home. I don't want an accident."

"Rest pretty lady. We'll stop soon. Want a cuppa up the road?"

"Yes. That would be good. I need a stretch. You probably do as well. We're making good time."

The break was what was needed. It was a hot day, with a vista of blue sky. They chatted happily and then soon headed north once more. They had stopped at Childers which was about another two-and-a-half-hour drive from their destination. This time, Jane was fully awake, and she strained more than what was necessary to make sure Mac kept his eyes on the road. The straight road.

Mac had to park the big home right up the back of the shopping centre in the heart of Tannum so that they were out of the way of other traffic and whilst he stayed with the home, Jane went and bought a few supplies and ice for the esky.

Soon they were at the holiday village without further mishap and the joy of meeting up and hugging family was the best medicine for Jane and Mac. It did not take long for them to set themselves up and with the grandkids excitedly checking out every little nook and cranny of the home, the laughter was spontaneous and music to the grownup ears.

"Let's go down to the pool, shall we?" asked Joanne once the parents were settled.

"Sure. Why not. Coming Mac?" Jane inquired.

"I think I'll give it a miss for now. Might have a kip. You go. I'll come down later."

The grandkids were more than boisterous with their love and wanting to show off their latest swimming skills. The water was cool and refreshing in the pool. Jane noticed dark clouds building to the west.

"Are we still going to the pub for dinner?" she asked the others.

"Yes. We are. We thought we'd go earlyish. We booked for 6pm. We can walk up. It's not far. Tomorrow being Santa day, the kids will have us awake at daybreak, so early to bed tonight for them. We might head back to the pub on Boxing Day for lunch. What do you think? We can book tonight while we are there."

"Sounds amazing. While we have plenty of food. It will be nice to be waited on for a change."

"How has Dad been?" Joanne asked.

"Funny you should ask that. We have had some interesting times. Remind me to tell you about his glasses later so that Tia can hear the story as well. I have to say though, coming up was a bit scary." Jane could not erase the look of worry on her face.

"Why? Traffic?"

"No. Dad kept driving to the left of the road. I was having a little nap and woke up suddenly with the noise a car makes when it travels continually on the white line. He was heedless of his bad habit. Got a bit shitty with me for suggesting he wasn't watching where he was driving. But all good after we had a break."

"That's not so funny, is it"? asked Joanne.

"No, it's not. It's scary. You try it. See if that doesn't make you sit up and take notice. I'll never close my eyes again whilst Mac is driving. I think he has a problem, but I don't know what it is!"

"Oh well. This week's holiday will be good for the both of you. I am sure you can relax. The kids are super excited to have you with us for a few days."

With that a crack of thunder that made them both jump.

Suddenly the day had turned to night as the storm started to sweep in with a bullying wind and eerie lightning and thunder. Everyone piled out of the pool. Grabbed towels and headed back to the camp site.

When Jane got back to the home, which needed the windows closed and the awning lowered, she wondered why Mac had not done that. Surely the sudden storm would have woken him.

She called out to him, but there was no answer. She busied herself in closing the home to secure state and then and only then, wondered once more where Mac could be.

Joanne's husband came to assist and make sure Jane was ok. He assured her that Mac probably had headed off to the loo and stopped somewhere to have a chat. Next minute Mac sauntered back and seemingly unperturbed of the building storm around him.

He stated he'd gone for a little walk and then added as an afterthought that he had trouble finding his way back to the camp site. He had to ask someone the way. He laughed as he opened the esky. Grabbed a beer and sat down in one of the comfy chairs they had brought with them. He looked at Jane.

"What's all the fuss. Only a little bit of rain. It'll be gone before we know it. Summer storms. You should be used to them hon!" he smiled at Jane.

Exasperation came close to release.

She said, "The home was open for all the world to wander in and live in. Thought you would have locked up before you took off."

"I never went far. Only over the road. All good. Want to sit and have a drink with me?" was his reply.

The worst rain in many years came in the next day and the next. Most of the tents, were all but washed away. Rivulets of water rushed here and there, causing mud slides and general disarray. It was obvious to everyone that they could not continue to camp.

A decision was made that instead of staying, as originally planned for New Year's Eve, they would head back to Joanne's home at Gladstone and celebrate there, where it would be dryer than the camp site. Mac and Jane said they would prefer to return to the Sunny Coast, as her house would have been bursting at the seams with everyone staying there. Mac stated that getting the motor home back to the dealership was a priority.

They did have access to the news and the weather predictions, but Mac and Jane were oblivious to the extent of rain that had been sweeping across the Queensland coastal fringe since Christmas Eve. They never realised they would encounter problems on the road, but heading south when they got as far as Childers, they were told that the highway was flooded, and that travel home would not be happening.

Putting in a call back to the Tannum Sands holiday place Jane and Mac were given assurance that they could come back and stay. It was a better option to sitting on the side of the Bruce Highway until such time as travel was safe.

Whilst a lot of the rain was further south of Gladstone, showers were present and annoying at times at Tannum. Still, it was pleasant enough. Mac and Jane managed a walk every day and a general relaxed state surrounded them.

If anything had evolved from the week it was the fact that something was not quite right with Mac. Jane was at a loss as to exactly what? He had been creeping around all week.

Mac had disappeared several times, then arrived back unannounced before any alarm bells could be rung. He never said where he went. If in fact he even knew where he wandered to.

He lost his new loafers. Every bin had been upended. Every little hidey hole in the home had been searched and he had no idea when or where he had last worn them. He certainly had worn them at the start of the holiday. They disappeared into thin air. Like the glasses and toiletries and the belt and the…and the…and the.

Jane approached the new year with a sense of foreboding. In her heart she knew her man was not 'with it' for twenty-four hours of each day. He was still the carefree spirit of old. He had lost none of his loving ways but there was a difference.

The statistics state that Memory Deficit during the first stage of Dementia is not evident. The individual could demonstrate any type of behavioural problems. There could be memory loss or confusion. Individuals without diagnosis are considered Stage 1 on the Global Deterioration Scale.

Dementia/Alzheimer's makes a difference to everyday lifestyle.

Mac was confused and he certainly had a small amount of significant behavioural problems. He was not aware of those behaviours. Jane on the other hand had it staring her in the face.

Mac maintained an everyday normal existence and unless Jane was watching and waiting every single moment of the day, which she wasn't at that given time, one would be forgiven for not picking up on anything untoward.

Probably in the carer's heart, there must be a point when they will realise more than the bloke next door, that all is not how it was, or should be with the individual suffering early-stage dementia. One must and can see silly moments creeping into a once normal day.

Whether that is noted or not, sadly, a lot of symptoms go undetected. Should an outsider suddenly notice an odd behaviour, they very rarely express their feelings out loud. Preferring to forget rather than make a big thing of it.

Jane remembered when Mac's sister and husband dropped in unexpectedly for a cuppa. The conversation flowed like it had done for many previous visits, but Mac did not join in as easily.

He seemed to struggle with some people's names. The moment was blessed with laughter, but his sister had not picked up his reluctance to offer his side to the story. Mac's conversation was different, Jane knew it, but she could not pinpoint exactly what it was at that stage.

Chapter 4 - Speculation and Contemplation

One of the many good aspects of their marriage, was the communication level. Also, they had enjoyed a healthy sexual coupling to that point in time. Jane was not a reluctant partner in the bedroom, but she was to realise that frustration had crept in with Mac and being able to offer what once he would have boasted to the world about.

She sensed his need, but more than once he failed to complete the act. This was a delicate situation for no male wants to be told he is a failure, and false bravado, and words of encouragement, do not appease all the time.

Jane and Mac were going away to celebrate a birthday at Hervey Bay. It had always been a good holiday destination for them. Easy access to clubs and pubs and because all walks were on a flat surface, Mac had enjoyed this exercise.

He mentioned in the week leading up to the holiday when he had an appointment with his GP for his regular B12 injection, that he might ask for some assistance in the bedroom, if he could get it. That was an eye-opener for Jane. Mac was obviously more worried about the lack of satisfaction in the bedroom.

Jane decided to go along to the doctor appointment with Mac.

She was observing, so to speak, as to what he did when he went to the doctor. He gave his name and details without any reason to be alarmed. The doctor was surprised to see Jane accompany Mac.

She said, "I've come to see what happens when Mac has his B12 injection. Who gives it, etc"

This doctor and Mac had a great understanding. A good rapport. They were about to leave when Jane prodded Mac and said, "Aren't you asking for something before you go?"

"No, what? Should I be?" Mac laughed.

Jane came straight out with it. She was a little tired of hedging. Said Mac was having trouble in the bedroom and that as they were going away for the weekend, a little help would go a long way. The doctor obliged, offered a once only pill and told him when and how to use it for best effect.

Mac didn't seem embarrassed. Neither did Jane.

The weekend weather was perfect. Longish walks. Swims in the pool. Dinner out. Drinks watching footy. The delicate bit was sex. When? How to introduce the little pill for best results.

Jane remembered all that was told. Obviously, Mac didn't. By the time the evening wore on and the idea of a cuddle before sleep might have jolted something in the memory bank, she asked had he taken the tablet as instructed.

"Which pill are you talking about?" He asked when questioned.

"The little blue one doc gave you, to help you in bed." Was Jane's reply.

"I took all my tablets this morning like I always do. You get them ready for me."

"Yes, I know but I didn't give that one to you then. Where is it?"

"Don't know. Must have swallowed it as well."

"It was sitting on the bedside table. I put it there to remind you before we got amorous to swallow it and wait for the fun to start!"

"Well, it's not there now, so I must have seen and taken it, thinking you forgot to give it to me with the rest of my pills."

Jane lay back against the fluffed-up pillows. "So, do you think you felt any different for taking it?

"Nah. Can't remember back that far. Can't even remember if I swallowed the darn thing."

"Oh well. If you did. Our walk was good this morning. And the swim later was good. Maybe you got a burst of energy in those things, hey?"

Mac looked suddenly sheepish.

"I'm sorry. I truly am. Have you had a good weekend?" he kissed her on the cheek.

"Sure have. It's been great!"

Jane knew in her heart, that pill or no pill, Mac was struggling with his inner self. He'd been a good lover. He had always looked after his Jane. Now, in that moment, he did not seem perturbed to turn off the light and go to sleep.

She sighed. What was happening in the here and now? She also made a promise to herself that she would not endure that experience ever again. It would hurt each other, she felt sure, yet she was more positive that it would hurt her more.

Then a couple of weeks before the next Christmas, Mac and Jane got invited down to his sister's place in Ipswich. His sister's husband was not well. Struggling with cancer and treatment.

It would not be a pleasant visit but one that was needed for both parties. His sister had always offered a solid hand of friendship since Jane and Mac had married. She had an easy acceptance of life and whilst the latest decline in her husband's health was test of endurance for her, she maintained a happy front to all she encountered throughout the ordeal.

Whilst Mac's daughter Marie, from his former marriage, was a breeze on a hot day, a laugh when the show was sad, a jellybean full of energy, his son, was the complete opposite.

Jane had nicknamed him the absent-minded professor. He always had his nose in a book whenever there was a get-together. He and Mac had not seen eye to eye since his marriage to Jane. Not that they were rude to one another, they did not gel like the daughter and him.

Jane learned they were to be visiting at Mac's sister's place. Mac was looking forward to the lunch and chats. It had been a while since he had seen both of his children, but he never got upset with any of the circumstances that surrounded their life.

Whether the extent of the long drive down, which on earlier occasions would have not been a problem, whether the prospect of meeting with his children did linger in his mind. Whether the fact his brother-in-law was bedridden, whether he was not being how he used to be, the day turned upside down.

Jane had no answer for the fact that within ten minutes of arriving, Mac had a funny turn. Funny as in strange. He lost his balance. He got all clammy. He sat down and stared into space. Jane got a cold washer and wiped his face. He sipped a little water. He did not talk for many minutes. He could not say a word to tell Jane how he was feeling.

It was horrible to watch.

After another good fifteen minutes, when he regained his composure, he was happy but a little more subdued. Quiet. His sister asked Jane if he had experienced these turns before. She questioned if Jane had mentioned it to the doctor.

Jane realised she must bring it up at the next appointment.

They had planned to spend the entire day with the family in Ipswich, but within an hour of arriving, Mac announced, because of his agitated state, that he wished to go home 'straight away'.

This annoyed Jane because she was unsure what was happening to Mac at this stage, and she was fearful that he may have another turn on the way home to the Sunny Coast.

He said he was tired and he slept the entire trip home.

The next morning. Mac seemed to be Mac again. Laughing and whistling. Jane asked him if he had a headache from his episode the day before.

"Why, should I?" was the question posed.

"I feel fine." was all he said.

Jane let it rest but vowed and declared on that day, she was going to make waves and get to the bottom of the ocean of unanswered questions. There was a reason that Mac was not well. There had to be, and whilst she shuddered inwardly that all was not well with her man, she knew she had to face those answers.

Stage 2 of Dementia suggests that signs of mild cognitive decline, also known as age, associated memory impairment, are common. Family members and caregivers notice forgetfulness from time to time, but memory issues may go undetected.

Names may slip a person's mind, or the individual may forget where he or she has left an object.

This stage does not warrant a dementia diagnosis and quite possibly signs of the disease would not be seen during memory tests. The person is still able to maintain and keep a job and participate in social activities. Bear in mind not all individuals with these signs will move on to the next stage in any set time.

Chapter 5 - Acceptance and Procedures

Within another few months filled with different moments, Jane became aware, before anyone else, that Mac needed a complete one on one interview with the lovely GP.

Firstly, the Christmas celebrations whilst they had been very lame in comparison to previous years, there had been several observances from Jane's point of view. She was not wanting to find anything wrong; it was a niggle in the back of her mind.

Mac had had another funny turn at work. The boss had rung her and asked if Jane could come up to Mac's work and pick him up. He didn't think he should be driving. They only had the one car. Mac drove it to work every day, except on the odd day that Jane might require it.

When she was confronted at Mac's workplace it was not hostile but real concern for him. He looked washed out. Was lying down in the area that was a designated, 'sick bay'. Jane talked with the boss. Discussed what she hoped was something mild, not a worry.

Jane said that perhaps Mac needed a more regular B12 injection. The boss shook his head as they talked. He did not want to alarm Jane, but Mac was having trouble at work.

He was not his usual self. The boss praised Mac in saying, 'he could sell rice to China if he had to,' but he was struggling with the paperwork and the other salesmen were not so happy to be doing it for him.

Righto. Jane got the picture. She assured him she would get some answers, talk further with his doctor, and go from there.

"Mac has a few days owing to him in holidays. Why not take them?" the boss suggested.

It could be the best medicine.

They headed to their favourite place. Hervey Bay. Now it had been four or five months since last there, and in that time, Jane was to discover a few odd pieces to the jigsaw of Mac's life.

The newest piece was floating. Jane was not sure where it would fit in.

Mac always packed his own overnight bag. She never questioned what he put in it. He only ever asked to select which shirt went with which pair of trousers or shorts. Jane usually laid them out on the bed, and he packed them.

The drive was sweet. No problems. They arrived at their regular holiday place, but for the first time in ten years, Mac had trouble finding his way to their unit. Did not seem familiar with the place, yet they always stayed there. Second floor, middle unit. Great views.

Between the two of them, which seemed to take forever, they did settle in, after which Mac was exhausted. Jane put it down to the long drive for they had not stopped at their usual place for coffee on the way up. Jane suggested a swim. Mac said he was going to have a kip before they walked on down to the pub for dinner.

Jane lay on one of the reclining chairs in the pool area. She must have drifted off to sleep. She woke with a start. Time had marched on.

Before returning to the unit the girl at reception called out to her. Did she know that the boot was open to the car, but no one appeared to be in or near the car?

Returning to the unit, Jane discovered Mac was in the shower. She asked him if he had been down to the car. Maybe? Why? Not sure. Keys? Not sure. Ok agreed Jane, she'd check it out.

She fixed up the car checked all was as it should be and returned to the unit. Mac was standing with a towel wrapped around him looking through his overnight bag.

"Did you not pack any undies for me?" he asked.

"No. You usually look after that. What did you pack in the bag, Mac?"

She looked. Folded neatly were the clothes she had laid out on the bed and other bits and pieces of clothing. No jocks.

Now Jane did worry at this oversight. Mac prided himself on two showers a day and liked to be cleanly dressed. Always. He had always packed most of his bag.

'Probably won't be happening anymore,' Jane decided.

She opened a bottle of her favourite bubbles. Rang the Thai restaurant downstairs and ordered take away. She got a beer for Mac and prepared to sit out on the balcony.

Before she settled herself, she went to see what he was dressed in. He had managed to pack his boxers that he wore to bed, and he had put a clean t-shirt on with them.

"I've got a stubbie for you. Come and watch the sun settle on the day!"

He did not question that they were not going out to dinner. Had he forgotten that as well. Perhaps the drive had been more than he was capable of? She asked if he had gone back down to the car. He replied he thought he went down looking for his undies. He shared that he thought he might have overlooked a bag and left it in the boot. Right! Moving On.

They settled in for a quiet night and enjoyed the Thai. The couple of days following went without mishap, but whilst they did a walk through the day down to the pub for lunch and collected some nibbles for later that night, Jane did not entertain a night out.

She guessed that might be stretching the friendship with her favourite man. She also offered to drive around for the few days that they stayed there. Mac was happy to let her.

The sad news that arrived on the way back home, was that one of Mac's favourite cousins, had passed away. The funeral was in two days' time. This cousin had been in Mac's life all through his boyhood and school days and later into their grown-up years.

The cousins had lived down the road from him, and they were affectionately called the three musketeers. Of course, it went without saying, that they would be attending.

That was a difficult day. One in which Mac's distant family of surviving aunts, and cousins and nieces and nephews, were privy to his forgetfulness. Mac had trouble remembering each of them, which he would never have experienced before. He did not seem secure in anyone's names, and before the day was over, he had inadvertently upset his sister, by his actions.

She had pulled Jane aside and questioned her, saying she thought her brother seemed different. He appeared forgetful; She reminded Jane that Mac's mother had passed away some years before and she had had Parkinson's related Dementia.

Now with that knowledge fresh in her mind, Jane booked another appointment with the GP. She was armed with thoughts and wanted answers.

Before Mac could get into to see the doctor, while they were in the waiting room, he had one of his funny turns. Perfect place for it to happen. Jane was to find out first-hand what they were. One of the trained nurses took him into a darkened room and he lay down for a little while.

The doctor joined them in there. He took his pulse, listened to his heart and everything seemed fine. Mac got up after about five minutes and went to the doctor's room. Jane quickly covered the previous week's events, leading up to and the other couple of times that her husband had had such a funny turn.

The doctor described it as Absence Seizures. They cause one to blank out or stare into space for a few seconds. They can be called 'petit mal' seizures. Apparently, they don't cause any long-term problems, however they can be set off by a period of hyperventilation. One may hyperventilate from an emotional cause such as a panic attack.

Jane could only think back and remember that Mac would have been overcome with excitement or even panicked leading up to them.

The other issue she wanted to address was that Mac's mum had Parkinson's Disease. She had noticed a slight tremor in Mac's hands, over previous months and it was increasing. Not at an alarming rate but it was defined.

The doctor did a quick test by which Mac stood up tall and held his hands above his head, but he could not hold them there for long for they started to shake. The doctor advised not prescribing anything at that stage. Said it was early days.

It appeared there was no medication for the Absence Seizures. If, of course, they became worse, more constant, then the doctor would look at further issues. Mac went home oblivious to what all had transpired at the doctor's surgery. He went to bed and slept like a baby and was a happy chap the next morning. However, he was hungry. Very hungry. He'd gone to bed with no dinner. A first for him in all the time Jane had known him.

Moving on from the instance when Mac had travelled to the left of the roadway driving to Tannum Sands, Jane was to discover that each time they set out for a walk around the coast where they lived, Mac once more preferred to walk to the left of the path and push her off at times until she told him to stop doing it. He, of course, was not aware he was doing it. She did wonder if this, too, was part of early Parkinson's. It certainly was an added worry for it had not been a habit in previous years.

The state of break down got worse after another month or so at Mac's work. The boss rang Jane again. He wanted to see her to talk over a few things. Now this boss was a good man. A very good boss and had had a lot of time for Mac. He was concerned to say the least.

The issue had come to light when Mac had had to shift a motor home and back it into another space. He could not get it right no matter how hard he tried. He sat down with his head in his hands and was visibly upset.

The boss had taken him aside and talked with him. They shared a beer but never spoke of the incident as Mac appeared to not know that he had had trouble of any sort.

When Jane went in Mac was surprised to see her. Whilst he went and got his work bag and collected his lunch things, the boss spoke quickly.

He said it was not the first time it had happened, but he felt Mac was a risk. He could not afford for Mac to pick up clientele in the homes and even taking them for a test drive would/could be a stretch. He apologised to Jane. He wanted to tell her before he broke the news to Mac. He was going to retire him.

OMG this was not what Jane saw coming at all. She knew in her heart Mac would not accept retirement. He was only sixty-five.

Stage 3 of dementia suggests that for people in the workforce, their performance may be impacted. Co-workers may notice that the individual may forget important issues that once would not have been a problem. Driving difficulties, poor organizational skills. Time management.

Jane could relate to all of this.

Mac had always been a reasonable cook, and it was his turn on a Thursday night, to surprise Jane and let her have a night off from the kitchen. In previous months, he'd not been half as exciting as a chef, and he struggled to put a meal on the table. The kitchen was left in a mess and the easiest of chores to be done, left undone.

Whilst dementia is usually not diagnosed during the third stage, the signs are important to recognise for early intervention. Furthermore, stage 3 may last for years. Some individuals may not develop stage 4 symptoms for seven years or longer.

Chapter 6 - The Fallout

"I'm not going to retire. Me? I don't think so. What will we do? What shall we do for money?"

All these anguished and volatile questions spewed out of Mac's mouth. He was insulted, to say the least that he had been retired.

He did not hold any grudge with his boss or the place that had kept him employed. He sat dejected. He was not whimpering like a baby but he was visibly upset.

"Why can't I work. I have to work. You don't understand. I'll not be sitting around idle." he cried in anguish.

It was a moment of despair. Then Jane was unaware in that moment that his next statement would have a far-reaching impact on them both.

Mac remembered a mate of his who used to work at a caravan place down the road from where he had been working. He decided he would go and ask could he have a job there. In his mind that was the solution to the whole mess of being out of work.

That led to the biggest upheaval to that date in Mac's life. Not only was the boss of this place a complete jerk and had little regard for his fellow man or work person, but he also abused Mac's intelligence and belittled him into believing that he was incapable of even being a good salesperson.

It is a given fact that caravan selling points are a little different to motor homes. Mac had to learn a few things regarding these sales. It was a whole new ball game. He tried very hard to understand the system. He had always been eager to learn. The fact that Mac was incapable of learning because of his condition, was a recollection much later realised by Jane.

On a very sad day not long after Mac had started work there, he went off to work at normal time. Within the half hour, he rang Jane. He was crying sitting in the car, he said. "I don't know where I am. Where am I going?"

"Oh Mac. You poor darling man. Have you any idea where you might be?" Jane asked concerned.

She got him to look around him. Make himself aware of his surroundings. Think where he could be going. It probably took a further ten minutes, then Jane rang him again and talked to him. She asked did he think he could find his way back home or would that be a problem. If it was, Jane would get help and get to him.

He had settled a little bit by the time he came home. Mac did not think it was the best idea at all. He worried about what the boss might say. He agonised over it, actually. He looked terrible. Washed out.

Jane suggested a shower and then a lie down. He slept for over an hour. Jane rang the horrid boss and said Mac was not well and would not be in that day. The boss abused her for the late call.

Said he would dock Mac's pay for loss of working hours. Said he would have to make it up over the next week. Jane decided there and then that Mac would never drive to that workplace ever again by himself. She was to take him to work for a further two weeks, in which the poor reception that Mac got at the workplace took its toll on him.

In the meantime, Jane went to Centrelink. Everyone needs Centrelink at some point in their life. It is not the nicest place to get quick results, but it is for the best most times.

She found out that whilst Mac was pension age, Jane was not and compared to what they would been getting, money wise, from the government, it would be a stretch. Mac had been getting commissions over the previous years. They could get rent assistance, if Mac took the pension, but there was a mile of paperwork and a lot of stuff had to be signed off by a doctor as well.

Jane sat down at the beach with a coffee. She realised she had to go back to Mac's doctor and have a serious talk. She was lucky to get in almost straight away with someone having cancelled their appointment.

He was surprised when he met her. He was even more surprised when he listened to the tale that Jane told of what had happened since Mac had been retired. He was as angry as Jane as to the treatment he was receiving at the caravan sales place. Jane asked for a referral to a specialist for Alzheimer's.

The doctor was not really in agreeance with that request. He doubted Jane's thoughts. He seemed to think that Mac was far too switched on to have dementia. Quite possibly the Parkinson's could be having an impact on his life, but that was early stages as well. Not something to fear, yet.

However, he reluctantly advised Jane of a recommended specialist and left it in Jane's hands.

Within another few weeks the first of the appointments with the specialist took place. Once more a mile of paperwork to add to the already growing pile of papers from Centrelink.

Finally, they both were to speak with the approved man of knowledge. They discussed daily issues. Jane did most of the talking, as Mac preferred to sit and wonder what was going on.

Never had Jane mentioned to him that she thought he could be bordering on dementia. She never used the word. Ever. The specialist saw Mac by himself and made his first assessment. Then he spoke with Jane.

He agreed that Mac had mild cognitive failure. He showed signs of possible early dementia, but he would not diagnose that until further tests could be done. He wanted a full MRI of his brain. X-rays and further blood tests. Meanwhile it cost the bleeding earth for all this. Mac had to have time off and that horrid boss was keeping a record of his time away from his employment.

Jane was getting more frustrated by the day not to mention how angry she was with life in general. No one person seemed to want to lend a hand and no one person that she spoke to about Mac's condition, namely his daughter and Jane's sister, believed there was anything wrong with him.

Within another two months, Mac had been officially diagnosed with Alzheimer's.

He had undergone a series of cognitive tests which he failed miserably. Jane had been questioned at length about every little aspect of what Mac did up to and including when he had come to the specialist's surgery.

A report was sent to Mac's GP, who in turn rang Jane and apologised to her for his failure to believe what Jane had been saying. He was still in mild denial. He simply believed that Mac did not display any real symptoms of Alzheimer's. He would take over now, though, looking after Mac and medicate him with appropriate medicines.

There would be no further advantage to seeing a specialist.

That doctor went on to help with appropriate paperwork and even advised Jane that she could apply for a 'carer's pension' because it was going to be impossible for Mac to work ever again.

Jane cried. She went for a long walk. She sat and could not stop the tears from falling. Who would she share this with?

When Jane spoke with Mac and tried to make him understand that he would not be going back to work, that he was officially retired, he sobbed like a baby.

"What's wrong with me. I'm perfectly fine. Fit and healthy, can walk and talk. Why?" He looked bewildered.

"Well, yes Mac, you seem ok but it will be best for us both if you don't work and who's to say we won't enjoy an early retirement."

Jane wanted to add, 'there is a lot wrong with you, but we'll get through this somehow. Someway.'

The pension came through after three months. It was nothing grand, but it was money. Jane's carers pension took longer but it was not something to write home about either. It was a pittance but with getting rent assistance, they paid their rent and put food on the table. There would be no more holidays anywhere of significance. Money would be a stretch.

Mac had been paying into a Super fund, but it had been eroded with fees as much as what went into it, and it did little to give them cause for celebration. Jane had long ago used her super fund to pay for Mac's hip and knee replacement operations. The well was drying up.

Still, they had each other.

Mac was her man, and he could be and was as loving as he had been all those years ago. Except in the bedroom. That had been brought to the attention of the specialist. He had asked Jane did she want Mac to have medication that could possibly help. She declined, saying it was easier to forget than remind Mac that he was inadequate in more ways than one.

The next issue that caused a lot of stress was that Mac had to hand in his driver's licence and not drive anymore. This was bigger than retiring. Jane had to make Mac realise that he was forgetful. He often forgot where he was going, in fact, had no clue how to get from point A to B; he solely relied on Jane to direct him.

He held her hand when he walked everywhere. They lived in an eight-floor apartment block. Their unit was on the second floor. Mac used to always take the rubbish down to the bins on the ground floor.

On more than one occasion he had gone up and down in the lift because he could not remember what floor they lived on and so never knew what number to press for the lift to stop. People in the block got to know and if he was seen wandering, they helped and got him back safely to their own unit.

It had been a' lightbulb moment' when Jane realised that the day Mac had been going to the caravan place and had got lost, she realised that all the time that her man had driven to the RV workplace that he had previously loved working at, he had done it basically by remote. He had been in his comfort zone. He knew the way. Timed it to perfection.

Take the perfection away and give him a new direction, he became lost and disorientated. He simply folded and cried like a lost child.

Mac always seemed happy enough. He often whistled a little of the same tune over and over. Probably stuck in his head. He tried to sing but had trouble with words. Jane had read that music along with exercise was recommended for preventing one's slip into more forgetful ways.

Their day was not like it used to be. It delivered something different from sunrise to nightfall.

Jane knew that Mac was happy with any type of music. It filled the unit where they lived day and night.

When Mac listened to music, he tapped his foot and his hands to the rhythm. The only show that Mac liked to watch on the tv was the footy and the nightly news. He had been an avid Broncos fan and he had been up there with the best with his tips. Whilst Sunday footy was still a stubbie and a pastime, that too was to eventually slide into forgotten dreams.

Mac never complained when Jane suggested a walk. He was often tired afterwards, but it filled up a few hours of a morning.

Stage 4 is moderate cognitive decline, where it is referred to as 'mild dementia' stage. When an individual enters this period, he or she will clearly demonstrate deficits when given cognitive examinations. An individual will show continued difficulties with concentration as well as recalling events.

Short-term memory issues may include forgetting what they have had for lunch that day or if in fact believing they have not eaten anything. Memories from past events may begin to fade or become increasing hard to recall.

The patient may find it hard to operate independently. They will have trouble with finances, and it will become harder for the person to be left alone, especially in unfamiliar areas. Social anxiety is common during this period. They may withdraw from social interactions because they have forgotten names of once familiar faces.

Denial about the symptoms will be become more relevant. They won't want to accept medical assistance. A care plan needs to be put in place and is highly recommended. The care giver may have to take over driving duties, and the patient then will need a lot of emotional support during this difficult time. This stage can last two years.

Chapter 7 - Decline and Assistance

On the same floor of the unit block where Jane and Mac lived, were an elderly couple who had been residing there for as long as Mac. They were always eager to accept sweet treats that Jane made and would often come in on a Friday afternoon and have 'happy hour'.

Jim and Jan were their names. Jim was a good talker and he delighted in swapping stories with Mac. He had been a publican out west around Winton and they had been managers of many holiday places over the years.

So, the tales were plentiful, and it passed the time. Mac had more spare time these days, because he and Jane were not socialising as much; these impromptu times were good for all.

That was the difference now. Plenty of spare time. Mac found it hard to go out. He never seemed comfortable around people. He said it was too busy out and about and it was obvious to Jane that home was where the heart was, and he relaxed more in his own comfort zone.

They did their daily walk and Jane swapped the walks around so that the scenery would be something of interest and a conversation piece. Sometimes, to make a difference, Jane would pack up the thermos of coffee and bake some sweets and she would drive them to another beach and sit and watch the ocean for as long as Mac was comfortable. Then they would do a little walk. She always knew that Mac would have a sleep in the afternoon, after this exercise, and it gave her a few moments to herself.

Her life had changed too. No longer the movie days with her sister. Her sister was not well either and Mac's sudden decline hindered those once easy conversations. Jane would find that if she was on the phone for any length of time, Mac would become a little hostile with her talking and he would start pacing, up and down the hallway of their unit.

Jane always had to ring off and put in any excuse not to talk on the phone for long. Her sister did not understand this. At all!

It made Jane angry that people did not get the situation as it presented itself. Not one person offered help in the here and now. She did not understand what was happening either, but her main concern was keeping Mac happy and quiet and not getting him upset.

The rest of the world whilst they might not believe her stories they had to fall by the way and wait for the day she had time to talk to them. If someone did not like her decisions. Too bad. So sad.

Jane had been told at the chemist where she got Mac's prescriptions that there was a home help service provided by the government, "My Aged Care". It varied in its assistance. Sometimes people can come to the house and sit with the person who was not well, allowing the carer to go out for an hour or more to do whatever.

Often these people could be engaged to help with the cleaning or shopping and be a companion for a limited time. Jane thought about this service; she did not need any home help. She was very capable of attending to all aspects of running the house. Instead, she realised that perhaps Mac needed some male company. He'd been associated with plenty of people over the years, maybe that could help with his unsettled mind.

Respite care also known as 'short-term care' allows carers to take a break from their care duties with peace of mind, knowing their loved one is being looked after by health care professionals. My Aged Care did an assessment of Mac and his habits and general living conditions.

There was very little lacking in Mac's care but what was enforced into Jane's mind was the fact, that the carer needs a life as well. The carer must keep going, regardless. They will suffer stress and burnout for the round-the-clock nature of caring for someone with dementia.

Additionally, many caregivers experience feelings of isolation, guilt and financial strain, amongst other challenges.

It was suggested that Mac could enjoy a couple of days a week at the Blue Care Centre. He would be picked up and returned home by bus. He would enjoy the company of people his age, and he would have a hot meal for lunch. There would be daily activities he could enjoy.

The daily ritual of Mac at this stage needs to be noted. He was, after many years of being an avid shaver not allowed to use a blade anymore. Too dangerous. Plus, his increasing hand tremors made shaving a delicate procedure.

Jane bought him an electric shaver. Whilst it never gave him the perfection that he always seemed to get over his previous shaving life, he was content to sit and use the shaver and be satisfied somewhat. He would sit for a long time. She let him. Small mercy.

Jane had to assist in the shower. Turning on the hot water and ensuring the temperature was right. That aspect had crept in overnight. Without Jane realising it, whilst simple, this was not something he could perform easily. At that stage Mac could still shower himself, take himself to the toilet when needed and could feed himself without too much trouble.

Jane always laid his clothes out on the bed each day, but he needed help with putting on t-shirts and tying shoelaces. One day he had sat confused as to how to secure his shoelaces. That was a sad moment. A proud man who had polished and worn lace up shoes every day of his working life. Jane helped him for several weeks before realising that shoes with Velcro fastenings, made life so much easier.

Jane made all Mac's shorts. It was easier to have elastic waist shorts rather than buttons and zips. Why confuse a situation further? He'd fumbled with buttons and left zips undone.

After breakfast Mac would take himself out to the front balcony and sit in his favourite chair and watch the world come and go. Their front balcony faced a very busy road. He got to say 'hello' to anyone who came down the front steps. He seemed content.

Sometimes he nodded off. Most times he would be idle, though he liked to mimic some bird's calls. Eventually after Jane had done the washing, or other household chores, they would share a cuppa and then she would take him for a walk. Lunch on return then a sleep.

The two days of respite offered a different routine. Up earlier. Showered and dressed before embarking on the short bus trip to the centre. Mac seemed to look forward to these different days. Reports came in from the beautiful, dedicated staff said that he was adjusting. He liked to have a sing-along. Did not participate in too many activities but if someone would help him, he'd always have a go.

At this stage Mac no longer walked down to the newsagent and bought a paper. Jane got up early, scooted down quickly and returned usually before Mac realised, she had left the building.

On respite days, she went when the bus had picked up Mac and took her time downtown with a coffee at the beach or a quick shop at one of the convenience stores. Mac no longer read the paper. He did not find that easy at all. He could not comprehend that concept.

On the days that he was home, Jane would read bits and pieces to him from the paper. She always completed a crossword and asked him continually for his assistance in helping her complete the task. Most times he chuckled and said that he didn't know or could not remember the answer, preferring to give her praise and say that she was the clever one.

As interesting as it is heart-breaking, unless Jane kissed Mac on the cheek, he would not initiate a kiss for her. He had stopped giving her a cuddle in bed at night. He did not offer any loving actions, except, he always called her 'his beautiful lady' and he always tried to whistle the same song to her.

Jane found it easier to do her main shop on Mac's respite days. Mac previously, when first retired loved to shop with her. He had managed Woolworth's stores in his lifetime, and he loved to look over the produce display and always had a chat with staff.

In truth it became easier, faster to shop without him. Mac could get anxious if they were with people for any length of time. Jane was always fearful of his Absence Seizures.

They'd hit out of the blue and she would be aware that he could not lie down in a grocery store whilst he came to and came back to reality. His actions leading up to these seizures were a trigger, yet Jane could not define what it was that set him off. She did partially guess that it could be anxiousness.

To that stage he had not had one of them at respite. She had made them aware what to expect if it happened.

Jane was Mac's constant companion. She never hesitated to try something different to make him smile. As a treat Jane might take him for a drive and pick up an ice-cream and go and sit at the beach and watch the waves for endless minutes. He liked the calming waves. He loved nature. He liked people watching. He never initiated a conversation. Mac tried to answer a question, if asked, but he never prolonged the sentence.

Jane and Mac had had their first trip on the Tilt Train to Gladstone. Previously they had driven there, but with the pension, one got a reduced rate in train travel. It had been relatively easy to set it all in motion. Mac had liked the trip. He loved the ever-fast scenery and he had not given Jane any undue anxious moments. Not sure he really knew where he was going but it was an uneventful trip.

Once at Joanne's place, Mac had days where he was at sixes and sevens, probably because the routine was different. He had been reasonable most days and had enjoyed the many different walks around their place. They had stayed for about eight days.

The children had been excited to see the grand-parents and had not noticed anything too amiss with Mac. The daughter had. The slowness of his gait. The length of an afternoon sleep. The not wanting to be sociable and go out to dinner. The biggest factor of that great holiday had been Mac's idea of doing something he had always done with pride.

Mac had always loved mowing. Joanne's husband did not seem put off by Mac offering to show the grandson, how that mowing was a great pastime and exactly how it should be done. It was so hilarious, yet sad, to watch.

Jane had had a bird's eye view from the top of the stairs overlooking the front yard. As Mac made a mess of the yard with no clear lines and absent-minded wanderings, the grandson looked on bemused. Once or twice, he took over from Mac and corrected the picture. Mac never did see the funny side to it at all. He believed he had delivered the best education in lawn mowing to his grandson and not a soul was going to say any different.

Noise levels were an interesting aspect of their stay. Mac hated loud tv, loud music or incessant children chatter even though he delighted in his everyday moments with the grandchildren.

Recalling this holiday in Gladstone prompted Jane to wonder how a few days with his own daughter might shape up.

Mac's daughter, Marie, lived down near Byron Bay. She asked Jane would she like to bring her dad down for a couple of days. Marie was concerned that Jane might not master such a big drive, and would the stay be too much for them? Once more Mac would be out of his comfort zone, and the forgetful moments were bound to be an issue.

To be invited down to Mac's daughter's place would be something different. A challenge. She did not have children. It would be quiet. Yet Jane prayed for a peaceful, few days. She really did want the daughter to see her dad and to see what she felt would have been a difference in his life compared to some twelve months before.

The drive was scenic, and Mac enjoyed it. Her place was comfortable, set in an enclosed compound. It was close to the beach so that was a bonus.

Walks each day to tire him out and a lovely chatty meal at night once the daughter had returned from work. The biggest worry was Mac not being familiar with anything around him. He did struggle with the bathing routine as the bathroom was nothing like he was used to at home.

He spent hours watering her garden which she loved and was grateful for. He surprised Jane after two days and asked when they might be going home. Not that he didn't like staying with and seeing his daughter. Far from it. They had a great relationship. He simply wanted to go home.

Jane suggested to the daughter not to take offence at their sudden departure. Which she didn't. If she saw any great difference with her dad, she never mentioned it and Jane did not push for an answer. Jane was happy that no major events had occurred throughout the stay.

The interesting part of that holiday was that many, many, times before, Jane and Mac would have driven to Byron Bay. They loved going down there because at that time, Mac and Jane had lived at Currumbin on the Gold Coast and it was always a great trip down the coastal strip for them and a pleasant day out at a different beach.

Jane used to swim in the bay, and they always took a picnic lunch. Mac could not remember a single aspect of the place. She had parked and they had walked around the beach area. Had lunch at the pub. Had wandered the shops and Mac remembered nothing. No recollection at all. It was sad. So sad.

One could be forgiven for never going anywhere ever again. Jane had reached the stage where she was trying to think ahead of Mac. Trying to envisage what he would do if confronted with something out of the norm. That was almost impossible. The individual who has been diagnosed with Alzheimer's, does not plan their day.

It is possible to prevent them from danger realising that they can't use the stove anymore because they can't regulate the heat or might forget to turn off an appliance. Those aspects are easy. They live in their world. One which has become their new comfort zone.

It may not be comfortable for the carer to watch this happen, yet the carer wants the day to run smoothly. Preferring not to be forever asking, "why did you that?"

The person suffering dementia won't give you an answer because they don't know why they do some odd things. There is no rule book to follow here. They are living a new life, and the carer must learn this life quickly to avoid the hours of frustration and anger.

Many, many times the carer will want to take back harsh words. To retract and not feel so bossy. That is a natural and normal instinct.

Each day a curved ball will be thrown. Learning to catch it will frustrate even a saint. Human beings do not set out to admonish every single action, but that aspect will creep in unless one takes the time to realise the patient is different.

Their world has changed, and so must the carer.

Chapter 8 - The Middle of the Tunnel

Whilst an individual with moderate dementia will have stages of severe forgetfulness, will need outside assistance, will have major memory loss, most likely will not remember his once 'off pat' phone number, they have moved along what is referred to as the tunnel.

By this stage he/she will be sitting in the middle of confusion and sliding towards harsher conditions, further frustration for the carer and awareness of not knowing what to do next.

The time of day being the most inconsistent aspect. Breakfast will not necessarily be at a given time. Sleeping in could change the colour of the day. Disorientation because of a fogginess from too much sleep will impact on the individual.

If days are planned, then the patient will accept with hesitance, time is of an essence. Not necessarily will they agree to all the carer wants them to do. They may well dig their heels in and refuse to have a shower.

To move at a quicker pace, the carer must think of a reason for changing up time. A happy reason. Not a 'we have to do this because' rather, 'if we hurry a little, we might get to go to the beach later and find some shells on the shoreline'.

Alternative living demands change as to how one thinks. The carer is thinking for two. The patient is not thinking at all. There will be many small arguments. It is inevitable. It goes without saying, the patient will find more reasons not to do something, than making life easy and doing it.

The carer will often remember back to how it used to be. How quickly the day's normality has changed and how the new changes can be absorbed, and make for comfort, not frustration.

Jane did not want to argue with Mac. She wanted peace. Yet, he seemed hell bent on making her day difficult. The 'witching hour'. The time before sunset. When night closes out the daytime peacefulness; where once Mac had enjoyed a sleep of an afternoon, suddenly he was restless. He did not want to lie down. Preferring to sit in his lounge chair and 'nod off' but not for long.

Where once he would have taken his medication without preamble, he now hesitated, questioning what the tablet or tablets were for. Not believing anything Jane said.

Mac said there was nothing wrong with him, so why take a pill. What was she doing to him. Trying to kill him!

Mac had a monthly appointment with his GP. General assessment. Fun talks and light banter. Only making sure he was ok. Checking on his Parkinson's. The doctor still believed it best not to medicate him for this condition. Believing that it would/could impact the tablets he had been given for his dementia disability.

Jane discussed at length that she thought that the initial impact of those tablets had worn off and that Mac did not seem to benefit from them as much as previously. The doctor agreed with some hesitance, believing that as the stages of dementia rolled through it would become harder to maintain pace with it.

There is no cure for dementia. Medication is trialled and whilst some may have some impact, they will not erase the condition.

The doctor suggested a mild sedative to help with a better sleep at night. Mac's tremors had moved to his legs at night. He was restless and not sleeping deeply like once before. Jane told him that he was being naughty and not wanting to take his medication.

The doctor laughed with Mac saying that he had a great companion in Jane, and it would be wise to do as 'the boss' suggested otherwise he may not get his treats for which Jane was able to create for him on a regular base.

Whether Mac comprehended any of this had to be seen to be believed. He was still angry at times for having to swallow pills, but he had pulled back on blatant refusal and at least thought about obliging Jane and doing what was asked of him. Especially if she presented a tasty slice or piece of cake on the same plate as the pills.

Jane and Mac had always managed a few days, from time to time in Brisbane with another of Jane's daughters, Tia. Her place over the years, offered a fun time, when they celebrated a birthday or special event. She had two daughters, who were very special in Mac's eye. He had a lot of time for them. They loved him immensely.

The next big event on the horizon, was Christmas. They were going to stay for a couple of days. Jane did not think it would happen without mishap, but she was keen to give it a go. She liked going down and staying there. She got to relax and have a few drinks and, being Christmas, even more festive.

Mac was good. He delighted in sitting out the back of a morning and using his electric shaver and would sit for as long as the battery lasted. It provoked laughter. Jane didn't care. He was happy. The other thing that brought much tittering, was that in the cool of the afternoon, Mac would sit and water the gardens and the lawn. He'd have a beer and lose himself in time. Jane was grateful for small mercies. She got to play Scrabble with her daughter, and it took the stress away.

They had a Christmas Carol event that went off without too much stress, and good food and wine blended with good company. All too soon they returned home.

For one little moment Jane had thought Mac was better. What prompted that thought was that they had not once had a harsh word.

It had been easy living with him. Sure, it had not been without a few instances but bearing in mind his surroundings had been different, and aspects of his daily routine, certainly changed, Mac had surprised even Jane's daughter. She found it hard to believe anything Jane may have previously confided with her.

Mac looked fine and behaved exceptionally well. Jane wished for more merry moments.

Those moments were a 'one of'. It was as though Mac had used up every bit of his nice manners. Had said every nice word over Christmas. The new year was set to change.

His first week back at Respite was terrible. He refused to get ready, and, in the end, Jane drove him to the respite home and cancelled the bus for the day.

Whilst he had a reasonable day, once there, he refused to get ready on his 'blue care days' in any hurried form. Then there was a bus trip one day, so she encouraged him and presented him with a new pair of shorts she had made for him, and he slowly made himself ready with her help and sweet talk.

Jane got a call before time was up that day because Mac had gotten sick on the bus and could Jane come and collect him. Mac had never suffered car sickness in his life and in the end, she realised he probably worked himself up to not wanting to enjoy himself.

He was happy to see Jane, it was like she'd been missing for a little while in his life. He had a big sleep on his return home and did not appear interested in dinner later. He seemed listless. She offered his favourite ice-cream and that was met with approval. Small blessings.

There were a series of Absence Seizures over the next few weeks. Random days. One of these happened at Respite. The first time it had occurred there. The staff were amazing, but it meant Jane had to once more collect Mac.

He could not travel on the bus. The same after-effects ensued, and the next day made for a more subdued Mac. They sat quietly on the balcony; he did not want to go for a walk. Did not want to have a sleep. Did not want to do anything.

Hours drag when a usual routine is disrupted. Jane had found an old photo album with many old pictures. That was a revelation for Jane but more hurtful was the fact that when she produced the pictures of when they had gone to Norfolk Island for their honeymoon, Mac had no recollection of any of it.

People and places that Mac should have remembered did not get a second glance and when she asked him to recall their last Christmas and the fun they had had at Tia's, his answer was vague. The words were sketchy and disappointing, to say the least.

Throughout the twenty odd years that Mac and Jane were to reside in the unit block, they saw a few changes in management. They were to meet a variety of people. Varying ages but most were middle aged or older. It was not a holiday rental property.

All residents were long term. It went without saying that people knew everyone coming and going. Of course, there were favourites and there were some that one did not get to know all that well for whatever reason.

One lady, Betty, was to become the 'mainstay' of Jane's life. An older lady, more like a maternal grandmother and mother figure rather than a friend. She had lost her husband sometime after Jane had lost her son. There had always been a connection between them.

Once, when Betty had been quite ill with the flu, Jane had taken up a cooked roast dinner with fancy trimmings, and desert to follow at her leisure. She had been ever so grateful. Preferring to stay within her closed doors for fear of spreading her germs, she was set to have a very lonely and quiet Christmas lunch. Jane had included her in her Christmas festive good will.

On respite days, Jane often took coffee with her. Offering treats to share. They talked amicably and Betty had many a story to tell. She had nursed her own mother with dementia. She shared some mind-boggling stories about the cunningness of the individual with this disease.

Betty never said at any one time, 'this is what will happen' rather, 'this happened, and it was so hard to understand and make people understand as well'.

That was what Jane was finding hard.

People's acceptance of Alzheimer's. Not many people believed half of the stories that Jane was to relate. Friends had dropped off many years previous; even family did not phone like they once did. Social activities had fallen by the way, because people were embarrassed by Mac's behaviour.

They did not know how to accept it. Did not know what to say. Jane felt like the 3rd wheel, if they had been invited out, because Mac did not offer conversation. Jane's life revolved around Mac and his new ways. She did not have any great stories to tell. She could only talk about her life now. People were conscious that Mac had become different.

When Jane and Mac had first been early residents at the unit block, Mac had been the life of the party. He always offered a tale, he was funny, he liked to share a drink and his behaviour was normal. Turn over ten years or more, he was a shadow of his old self. Yet Betty understood. She calmly settled into Jane and Mac's life without being in their face. Jane was to realise she needed her. She needed her more than what was obvious then.

Mac's brother-in-law passed away with cancer complications. It was a sad moment for all the family. Sure, Mac realised for his sister's benefit that she had lost a loved one, but throughout the service it was obvious that Mac was struggling and almost to the point of asking what they were doing at the funeral home.

There was the usual wake and whilst people came together and offered a host of stories, Mac did not want to partake, and this was a glaring omission. Mac would have always had a story about his brother-in-law. They had been good friends as well as becoming related. He was sad when people hugged him. He cried with them, but Jane was pretty sure he did not really know why he was crying.

Episodes of confusion were becoming more commonplace.

Mac had lost his way on his way down in the lift if he got out of the unit, without Jane's knowledge. She had to ensure the unit stayed locked, to stop him from wandering outside that door.

Outside the unit, to the left was a fire stairwell. Jane was fearful if Mac was to get in there he would not get out. May fall, even hurt himself.

She had become more vigilant and aware that the middle of the tunnel was no place to live in.

Chapter 9 - Severe Cognitive Decline

"Mac what are you doing?" Jane's voice was a little sharper than usual. Perhaps it had been a rough week.

Mac was in the shower with his clothes on. There is a funny side to dementia. Not everyone would think that, but Jane was to discover that several actions of the patient, make sense in their world.

Jane had laid Mac's clothes out on the bed as a normal routine.

He had gone to the toilet before he was to take a shower. Something in his mind closed and he stepped into the shower fully clothed when she had left him to his morning personal ablutions. She had wondered what it was that had made him do this. It was a first.

"Mac, you have your clothes on, hon; you can't wash yourself like that!"

"I'm saving you a job." He replied unperturbed.

"How's that?" she asked.

"You said you were going to wash the clothes; I'm helping."

Jane sat down on the bed and looked at Mac take his time rubbing soap into his clothes and letting the water wash the suds through. Oh dear!

She had bought a shower chair for safety. Mac's tremors were increasing, and it was impossible for him to stand that long in the shower for there were no handrails in the shower recess.

She'd read only a week previous, a very interesting book on the developments of dementia and some of the issues that present when the patient's mind slides off the Richter scale and settles in the slush field of mush.

The woman who was telling the story was relating how her mother had forgotten what to do in the shower. She had had to stand outside the door and go through the motions and watch her mother try to mimic her inside the shower.

Up to this point Mac could shower himself. Whether it was as good as the previous ten years, one would have a point to argue, but general showering care is a personal issue, and some people will take offence when the carer suggests they might need help. Jane was not looking forward to that day. For now, he was happy to shower without aid, though he needed help in drying himself.

When Mac realised what he had done. He laughed and said, "Oops!" took off his clothes and added, "they're clean now!" Then he proceeded to soap himself.

There was little point to admonishing the action. Mac did not see anything wrong in his mind. He was simply helping do the washing. Somewhere in his mind he had heard Jane say, shower and washing. He connected the dots and went about the task.

Jane was to learn that too many words in too many sentences confuse the poor, deteriorating brain. She had had to adjust her ways and speech. Keep it simple when making a statement. Less words better impact. Make repetitive requests, quietly, and keeping a request simple will hopefully ensure best results.

Jane was to learn the hardest element in looking after Mac was, 'Don't preach. Don't screech!'

It is almost an instantaneous retort when the patient does not do what the carer has asked of them. They chastise for lack of understanding. They admonish for lack of hearing skills.

A favourite of Jane's was "Are you deaf? Did you not hear what I only said a minute ago!"

Carers will continually get frustrated when the patient sits and stares into space with little comprehension of the last few words uttered to them. By no means should the carer feel that they are being unsympathetic to the patient's demands.

It is a natural element to be as frustrated as the patient. Yet, one must learn to curb the urgent instinct to retaliate and follow it up with a good reason.

"Seriously. Mac. Don't do that, please."

"Why not!"

"Because you could get hurt. Then, that would be terrible."

As the natural gait of Mac declined, his spatial awareness went out the window as well. The walks every day were now not as long. Without Jane keeping her man confined to the unit, Mac would have stumbled unheeded down the road and been run over at the first crossing, if he even got that far. Jane had to hold his hand tightly and refrain him, like holding back a little toddler hell bent on discovering a new world.

She found his footsteps sluggish for he was walking as though the ground uneven. He would stumble if Jane did not tell him to lift his feet a little. When she came to an intersection, she would have to tell him that there was a slight drop down from footpath to roadway. He never wanted to stop, look and listen. Wanted to sail forth without a care in the world.

It had been six months since they walked on the beach. The beach that Mac loved. The ocean with its calming, whispering, voices falling into the mind, to steady it.

The sand became too uneven for him to walk on without a stumble. The other interesting aspect was that he wanted to walk further and further out into the ocean, by himself, preferring not to hold Jane's hand. He would not stay on the shoreline and let the gentle ruffle of shore breakers keep his feet cool.

Jane did not wish to have to continually tell him to come back out of the water. The beach is a pleasant place, but those walks were starting to become a problem and as much as Jane could lose herself there, she was often on edge worrying about Mac.

Their daily walks were also becoming exhausting for Mac. They preferred to rest more in the shade of the trees at Happy Valley having a coffee. Jane always brought a treat to eat with it.

Still, it was fresh air. It filled in time and even if her heart was in her mouth some days when Mac did some silly things, she reminded herself he did not really know he was doing them.

The old Mac would have been horrified with his antics. The old Mac was gone, and Jane had to get on with the new life, with her new Mac.

Jane was to discover that when they sat out the front on the balcony with a coffee or lunch or crossword or a general connecting time, Mac would never start a conversation. Always staring into space. Listening to the general rush of life around them.

Jane wondered what he was really hearing. If prompted, he would respond but that was not a given, either. Not that long before Mac would have liked to talk about his days when he had managed a Woolworths store out at Charleville.

Now Jane would look at the Woolworths ad in the paper and make a comment on food prices or something, hoping for a quick jolt to the mind. Sadly, now she only got monosyllables.

It had been one of the happiest times of his life. His daughter had been two years of age and his son had been born out there. He and his first wife had made good friends. It had been hard for them away from family, but he had obviously made the most of those living conditions and work commitments.

There were many such tales about his early selling days as a car salesperson. He had roamed around and had met many interesting people. Jane always prompted to get a story, hoping, but he was tired within minutes. It was like he drove the miles through the years.

Jane asked Mac daily to remember his name. He would say it with conviction giving himself a full title. He did not have a mobile phone anymore to remember that number, nor did he remember the home phone number. He knew his address but not the unit number. Jane had given him a bracelet which was inscribed with his condition and their phone number on it for his sake and if he ever did wander away, someone would help him return.

Jane had read also, that some individuals will demonstrate compulsion like repeating behaviours. He or she may want to clean the same thing repeatedly. Mac wiped the bench down each morning at least ten times. There was not a speck on it, but he was happy doing that chore. The other annoying habit was he wanted to pick up things off the hallway carpet. Obviously in his mind he could see something and continually bent over and pretended he had found a thread or small article.

Joanne, who lived in Gladstone had had serious back problems. She had been to Brisbane for an operation and was returning to her home, but she needed extra care. Not allowed to drive for a few weeks. General conditions, for her and the family, at home, would be compromised.

She hated to ask considering how Mac was progressing through the tunnel, but she asked anyway. Would Jane come up and stay and help with the kids and general household duties. Her hubby was a fly in/fly out worker. He would not be around to help twenty-four seven nor would he be home for long when he did get his break.

Jane did have to think seriously about the request. The fact that Mac loved going to Gladstone and being with Jane's family, swayed her into believing that she'd give it a go. If it got too much, she'd return home to some sort of normality as soon as she was able.

The previous trips on the Tilt Train had been a pleasure. This time presented a few problems that had not been there before. Mac was restless. There was a noisy family with a toddler a couple of seats away.

Jane had noticed noise levels were something that made Mac get agitated. Mac spoke loudly more than once asking, "Can you shut that kid up? I want to sleep!"

If there was something that Jane was guilty of, it had to be, being embarrassed for/with Mac and his outbursts and moments. He looked normal. He appeared with it. Yet his angry outbursts, especially when he raised his voice, were frightening and not something Jane was to cope with all the time.

Sure, up until now, she could quieten him down at home, but out in public, she demurred. She touched his arm. Quietly letting her hand trail up and down his arm. Saying soothing words and trying to tell him that it was public train, and they were not the only passengers. He put his head back and rested. Eventually he slept.

Not one to let a moment slip by Jane got up and went and spoke to the mother of the naughty child. She apologised for Mac's outburst. Told her that her husband had Alzheimer's and that some days were hard for him. He meant no harm.

The woman looked at her like she was an alien. Muttered something rude and turned her head back to doing whatever with the brat. Jane felt it was really that woman who should have been apologising for the unruly child, but she let it go and tried hard to not let the incident get the better of her.

Then Mac decided when he woke from his snooze, he wanted to go to the toilet. That would not have been a problem previously. He could deal with that. Except now, he certainly had problems getting his feet to work with the motion of the train.

It was a trial for Jane to get him to the loo and wait outside, with the door ajar, whilst he attended to his need. As everyone knows there is very little room in these cubicles. She prayed he'd be able to carry out that quick pee. She prayed he would not embarrass himself or her further by wetting himself.

Something of note here and it is delicate, but a normal procedure, in the scheme of things changing in the patient's life. Mac could no longer stand and pee. He had had to sit down and get on with the job that way.

That had been a learning curve that had presented at Respite.

One day, he had gone about the usual task only to realise his aim was not good with trembling hands and he made a nice mess of his lovely shorts he'd been dressed in. Not to mention his clean shoes. Staff had been wonderful. Jane had had a lesson in showing Mac what to do from that day forward. She'd bought a 'chair over commode' and it fit nicely on the existing toilet in the unit.

Right at that moment, on the train travelling fast to Gladstone, Jane wished for it to have wings. She wanted out of this scene. *Change it up, please! Quickly*! She prayed to herself.

This trip was also a turning point. They were far from their comfort zone and suddenly, these everyday moments away from that scene, seemed to Jane to not only be an added trial, but one of a huge effort for Mac. One can only imagine what the patient thinks, but Jane was to realise, the patient does not think like the norm, or how they once, normally did. They set the scene to suit their needs and if the carer is not up with script writers, the carer is left behind learning the lines.

Jane had never been so glad to see her daughter. It was impossible to share all of what had happened on the train. That noisy family had disembarked at Bundaberg, so the trip on from there had been uneventful and quiet. It was, once more, great to be with family.

The effect of living away from home did have more moments of realization than previous. Mac had never wanted to go to the loo through the night. This time he did, every night. Jane had to make sure he could find his way and whilst that had been a new thing, settling him down again was hard. It was almost like, 'let's stay up now! I'm awake. I'm hungry.'

His morning shower presented further issues. Joanne's house was a rental through the education system. It was on the oldish side. It did not have a modern bathroom and the shower was over the bathtub. Jane had to help Mac into the tub to shower. Ensure he washed himself with the minimum of fuss and help him out once more then dry him. This extra new routine was enough to wear him out. Not to mention how wet Jane could get herself in helping him.

The electric shaver had been a great new toy for Mac to play with. Suddenly he decided it didn't give him the close shave he desired. He wanted to use a razor. Jane decided to play a new game with him. So, with fear and trepidation she learned the fine art of getting rid of his whiskers, with a razor every morning.

The biggest hurdle was that Mac had to agree she had done a good job. He would sit rubbing his hands over his chin and face. He praised her. Thank heavens. Whilst she was at it, she bought some hair clippers and started giving him a two blade. He looked like a new man.

The usual walks around Gladstone that the two of them had entertained on previous trips, became arduous. There was a lovely coffee place at a lookout not that far from Joanne's place.

Mac had always enjoyed that walk. Jane was to learn it had become far too much for him. They only did it the once. He was exhausted. A couple of smaller walks were still in the offering, but Jane noted he looked for his afternoon nap once lunch had been consumed.

The noise levels were an ongoing issue. Mac would go to bed before Jane. She liked to sit up for a little while watching something of interest on the tv or talking to her daughter, and letting the day's events wash over her and prepare her for another day. It was nice to not have to constantly be watching Mac and keeping him safe.

Those moments were short lived. Mac started yelling at her to come to bed. Said the tv was loud and needed to be turned off or down. It was easier to appease his requests.

Jane seemed never to win an argument when Mac was strong in his belief that his word was law.

Instead of returning on the tilt train, which Jane had confided caused a few problems, it was decided that as Joanne had an appointment with the back specialist in Brisbane, they would drive back down to Jane's unit. She would then proceed to that appointment after a day or two. The kids would stay with Jane and Mac as an added treat.

Jane did not see anything wrong with this arrangement, but she knew it would be hard on her daughter sitting for that long in the car. They would have to share the driving. It would have been better to take a quick air flight. However, she agreed.

Joanne had responded well to rest and could feel an improvement with her previous back issues. The trip back with all the family was two-fold. Mac was having a birthday. A special seventieth birthday and they wanted to be there for it.

Yes, it had been ten long years since the wonderful happy celebrations of his sixtieth milestone. What a lot of water under the bridge since then! There would be no big celebration at a club or pub. They were going to have lots of lovely food and drinks at the beach not far from the unit that Mac and Jane lived in.

BBQ sausages, chicken and salads. Most of the family and grandkids were coming. Mac's daughter and son and his little girl would be attending. The only friend of Mac's to attend was

Betty. How sad that all the friends had dropped off the radar. In that short time, life had indeed changed for Mac and Jane.

It was a pleasant day. Mac tried to sing along with anyone who prompted him into doing so. He whistled a few bars of his favourite song, laughed with the grandkids and managed to eat a good amount of food. He seemed to know everyone. Or was he pretending? He nodded and smiled throughout the day.

The sad ending to the day came later. On returning to the unit, there were a few family members present. Betty came back and took pride of place at the table of celebration. They were going to cut the cake. Suddenly, Mac decided he wanted to have a sleep. Jane suggested a shower instead, to help himself feel fresher.

Jan and Jim who lived on the same floor as them, were coming in for cake. They said they would not attend the beach party but would love to share a special 'happy birthday' with Mac on his return from the day's activities.

Joanne's kids settled themselves in front of the tv with a movie. The noise level was not through the roof, but it was probably above the normal.

Jane could hear Mac shouting out from the bedroom. She'd put a clean set of clothes out for him on the bed. She went in to see what all the commotion was about, and to help him dress. He was very abusive to her. Wanted to know what was going on? She told him quietly that he was going to have cake with his friends.

He yelled at her, saying that he didn't need people coming into his house, making noise and running the show. He had rights, you know. Didn't he? Jane tried to settle him telling him it was his birthday and that people wanted to share his special moment. Before Jane could get his clean t-shirt on him, he opened the bedroom door and stormed down the hallway.

"What do you think you're all doing in my house. Go home the lot of you. I've had enough of this noise!"

The children looked frightened. The adults looked stunned. This was the man who had sat and enjoyed his day at the beach. Jane took him by his hand and sat him down in his favourite chair. She got him a cool drink and dear loveable Betty came and sat beside him and calmly said,

"What a great day, Mac! I haven't had any cake yet; would you like some with me. I think Jane has done an excellent job again with baking you her best cake yet!"

"Who's Jane?" he asked putting his head back and resting his eyes.

"Your wife, of course." Said Betty.

He opened his eyes and looked at Jane standing in front of him. There was little recognition. There was no smile. Betty indicated for Jane to move away, all the while she kept up a gentle conversation with Mac.

He settled and slipped into a doze. She still talked to him sensing that he could hear her. Jane made herself scarce. The parents had taken the kids out to the front balcony and were quietly reflecting on what had happened to bring the day to a sad conclusion. Jane joined them. She did not want to cry. She did not want the kids to fear their grand-dad, but they had to be told that sometimes grand-dad forgot where he was and who he was, and that we all had to learn to live with it.

The day closed without any further yelling or gnashing of teeth. The guests went home.

The next day Mac was Mac again. Although somewhat subdued. He had a quiet belated drink with Jim in the afternoon. Jim who made no comment, only to say, "What's happened to our Mac, Jane?"

The family finally returned to Gladstone within a few more days. No one really wanted to say much about any of it, but Jane knew that maybe the day had been too big for him, tipping him over the edge!

Plus, Jane realised that Mac was not the drinker he used to be. He still enjoyed a stubbie, but he sat on it for longer than once would have been possible. Mac had had a few more than his normal intake.

During this severe cognitive decline, the individual will have trouble communicating. Emotional issues are very common. Short bursts of vindictive and spiteful words will ensue. The patient will often become agitated and more delusional. Sleep patterns are impacted with sleeplessness at night creeping in with what would have been peacefulness in the months and years before. If the patient suffers at night, it will result in exhaustion throughout the next day.

Sometimes the individual can become very agitated, and violence can occur in an otherwise non-violent person.

During this sad stage which can last two and three years, incontinence becomes an issue with the individual having difficulty with controlling their bladder.

Chapter 10 - A World to Live In, One to Be Believed

Where did the loving moments of two people flee to? Why did he decide overnight that Jane was not Jane at all? Why would the brain suddenly lose that vital bit of stored knowledge? To slide off into the slush field and wallow in the abyss. The one that had grown daily for the last few years.

Jane was more than aware that noise was an increasing factor. The tv very rarely went on. Mac preferred music and she did not resent listening to that with him, at all.

New daily habits were a stretch. Mac continued to go to respite two days a week. On more than one occasion he would have one of his Absence Seizure moments and Jane would have to go and pick him up and bring Mac home. A sleep ensued. He very rarely remembered he'd been to respite, preferring not to talk about his day.

Over the Christmas holiday break his daughter and husband had come up for a couple of days. They kept to themselves and were little hindrance to Jane. Mac recognised and knew his daughter and her voice. He delighted in seeing her. He loved her.

Yet, on one night after he had been for his usual afternoon nap, he demanded who the people were in his house and if they were going to stay then they needed to be quiet. He'd not been like that since his birthday some weeks before. Tolerance and space. His space. Not wanting to share anything.

The once long afternoon sleeps had diminished. He was napping. He was restless. His agitated state on lying down probably hindered him from slipping into a comfortable sleep. The saddest event was to shake Jane to the core.

They had been resting one afternoon. Jane was reading lying beside Mac. He'd not slept long and when he woke, he was grumpy and agitated. Jane tried to appease him.

"Who are you to tell me what to do?" he yelled at her.

"Shush! Mac don't yell. Lie back down a few minutes and I'll get you a cold drink."

He looked at her oddly. Comprehension was not present.

"Where's my wife?"

"I'm here Mac. It's Jane!"

"You're not my wife. You'd better leave before she gets back."

Jane did not know what to do. The first time that Mac had physically rejected the idea that she was his wife. She became as agitated as him. She yelled at him which made him worse. She repeated who she was, but he refused to back down from his rude words, and as she was to get up off the bed, he pushed her down.

"Find my wife, I tell you."

Jane went out to the kitchen and rang Betty. Told her what was happening. All the while she could hear Mac yelling out on the front balcony. Yelling out, "Anyone seen my wife!"

Oh, dear, what to do. Betty suggested she hide in the laundry and let Mac do a little rant and see what happened from there. She did this. Mac was hell bent on walking up and down the hallway by this time, starting to sob and pleading with no one in particular, to help him find his wife. He eventually went and sat in his favourite seat in the lounge room.

Jane was on the mobile phone to Betty. She suggested she give Mac a few minutes to calm himself then appear before him, change her clothes and try and settle him.

Jane pretended that she'd been outside and came into the lounge room and asked Mac what was wrong. He started crying. He recognised Jane. He said he thought she'd gone away. Did she go away? She replied that she'd been in the shower and heard him yelling and wondered what was wrong with him. He did not seem to think he'd been yelling. He'd denied it.

She made him a cup of coffee and got some of his favourite slice and they sat together in the lounge. He rested his head back and dozed. He looked terrible. Washed out.

Jane was washed out as well. Sour on the world and everything in it. Never had he turned on her. Never had he not known her. There had been the incidence on his birthday when he had questioned who Jane was, but it had not led to anything like this.

Jane was not fearful, yet, of his actions. She doubted Mac would hurt her. However, she was not to know then, how fearful, and tearful she would become with the incoming events.

Jane made an appointment for herself with Mac's doctor. He suggested a mild sedative. It might help. Not only could it be used at night-time, but if Jane felt Mac was going to get a bit 'iffy' with her directions, or how Mac was behaving, she could give him the medication. It would calm him. Maybe.

Everything with Mac was a trial. One never knows what medication will help until some results may appear. She had a long talk with the doctor. Jane cried for the first time whilst she related what had happened. He could sympathize with her for the road had become very uneven.

The doctor assured her she was doing more than was necessary. He suggested that there was care available. Jane demurred once more. She was not ready to let her Mac go. She'd never entertained that thought at all; believing she was quite capable of looking after him.

Within the next week Mac once more refused to take his medication. Said that Jane was trying to poison him. She used the doctor's name and said that he would be upset if he thought that Mac was being deliberate in not wanting to take his medicine.

"Prove it. Get him on the phone!" Mac yelled.

She did try but as anyone knows, doctors are busy, very rarely do they take home phone calls and with the receptionist telling her that she would pass on the message, Jane had little reason to be happy with the situation.

Jane tried a different approach, she rang Mac's daughter, thinking she might be able to persuade him to be good. He talked with her for a few moments, but never did he agree to swallow his tablets.

Another call to Betty, was the only answer. She came down within a few minutes. Having made some pies for herself and Betty for dinner, she had come to collect her share. She talked with Mac in her usual quiet voice, and he listened.

She noticed Mac's medication sitting on the bench. Betty asked him had he forgotten to take them. He never said yes, or no. Jane told Betty that Mac was being naughty and not taking his tablets, and like the naughty boy that he was, when Betty offered them to him with the assurance that he would feel better for doing it, he swallowed them without preamble.

Jane could only sit in wonder.

Sometimes the carer is the worst enemy. The hidden threat to the everyday life that has been reached. If Jane had been told it was not intentional for Mac to treat her with disrespect, she would have taken little reassurance from such words. Jane could not comprehend how Mac could/would suddenly turn on her. Why?

She knew he loved her. Why would he treat her like he did?

Over the next few months, Jane's patience, love and tolerance were tested beyond belief.

There was one night, one horrible night. Remembering the witching hour that Jane had read about, sometime before dark and usually after an afternoon nap.

Jane, this time had been at wit's end as to what to do.

Mac had yelled and screamed at the top of his lungs out on the front balcony, asking all the world to find his wife. Once more he had not recognised Jane. He kept his tirade up for some time. One neighbour came and knocked on the door. *Could they help? Mac seemed distressed. Had Jane been out and left him by himself?*

Jane had replied she had been there all the while listening, nothing she could do or say would change his tune.

"Do you think we should call an ambulance?" the neighbour asked.

"What for?" was Jane's reply.

The neighbour suggested that maybe they could take him to hospital. He might need some medication.

Jane waited for an hour before the ambulance arrived. Mac had sat out on the balcony crying and yelling out, then had finally come into the lounge room. Exhausted.

The neighbour talked with him quietly before the paramedics arrived. Jane made herself scarce. When they finally arrived, they were amazing. Helpful. They talked with Mac. Took his pulse and blood pressure. He was fine. Not having a heart attack or seizure or anything other than being demented.

One of the paramedics knew firsthand what Jane was going through. His mother had had dementia. He suggested that Jane should really look at getting permanent help for Mac.

"Thanks," she said, for the tip.

Jane had gone downstairs to bring up the paramedics into the unit. In the short time that Jane had disappeared and returned, Mac remembered who she was, and he was not as volatile or abusive whilst the professional people were there.

They could see little reason for Jane calling them out, because his moment of madness had worn itself out. They did not admonish her for her actions though she felt foolish and embarrassed to say the least.

It had been then that the lovely paramedic had told her about his mother. He knew what Jane was going through. His mother had done the same to his dad. Daily.

When these abusive sessions started to take place daily, Jane would often take herself downstairs. Sometimes Mac could be appeased quickly but that was not a given. These rants took at least fifteen to thirty minutes to subside. She'd ring Betty and Betty would come down and sit with Mac. He always knew her.

After a time, enough time to allow Mac to sit quietly with Betty, Jane would return up to the unit. She'd pretend she'd been out for a walk and Mac was happy once more to see her. There was little point in preaching at this point.

If Jane was not Jane, there was no way Mac was going to listen to her. She was a nobody. That hurt Jane immensely.

Chapter 11 - Severe Dementia

There are more than 100 types of Dementia, with Alzheimer disease being the most common, followed by Vascular dementia, Lewy Body disease, and front lobe dementia.

Stage 7 is considered the final stage on the global deterioration scale. Usually, the patient will lose the ability to communicate effectively. Angry outbursts are more widespread as the individual feels extreme agitation. Sometimes this stage can last upwards of two years.

These abnormal bursts of anger, that Mac suddenly developed, did not always follow the same script. Sometimes the moments were weird. Mac would swear someone was coming out of the walls and threatening him. He would tell Jane that they were real.

She knew he was hallucinating. Sometimes he'd hide in the shower. Preferring to sit in the darkness until such time as the demons went away. Those type of scenes were not all that often. Most delusional outbursts were when Mac did not know Jane; resented her being there, and they offered more challenging and difficult times for her.

On some afternoons, and even night-times, when Mac would suddenly decide that Jane was not Jane usually the help of Betty soothed his ruffled feathers and peace would reign again. Jane was to ask the staff at respite if he ever got angry there. There had been no incidence thus far, but they did confide that he never wanted to join in activities anymore and preferred to sit and listen to music and snooze in a comfortable chair.

Some nights when Mac was getting restless and agitated with not knowing who Jane was, she would not chastise him for his slip in memory, preferring to take Mac by the hand, put on his walking shoes and take him for a walk around the block.

All the while she would talk to him asking him if he thought he could see his wife. Did he think she'd be out for a walk or maybe she could be home waiting for him when he got back. She never left the building without telling Betty. Betty would stand out on her balcony and watch them walk around the block. She'd be waiting for them on their return.

She'd then look to Jane for clarification as to whether Mac was with it or not. Depending on this, Jane would sometimes make herself scarce and Betty would bring him back up to the unit. When Mac saw Jane, he'd be so pleased and usually cried on her shoulder, fearing she had gone away again.

Jane realised that these latest happenings in their life could not continue. She spoke at length with Mac's daughter and her own daughters. They had been kept up to date with the decline in their father's life, and they wanted her to get a relief respite package and have a little restful break herself whilst he would be in care. Jane declined.

Having always maintained that if Mac was to go to care, then it would be for a permanent stay. Not a holiday. He would never adjust during or after. Jane was almost sure of that. His decline was increasing, and she was clinging to some little bit of normality.

There was something that Jane wanted to do. Mac and Jane were going to be celebrating twenty-five years of marriage. That was a milestone and Jane wanted it to be special. She wanted to go back to Hervey Bay. The family offered to pay as part of a gift to them. It was a holiday destination that they had both loved and it might be good for Mac.

Those few days were happy and sad. Not once did Mac remember anything about the resort that they stayed in. He did appear to recall the view out to the ocean when they sat on the balcony although he insisted on saying it reminded him of another time, somewhere. The walks that they managed were gentle and nothing like previous times.

Jane took the car down to the pub which had been a favourite eating place, and in those days gone by, within walking distance.

They sat quietly eating their meal and after a little drive around the esplanade returned to the unit. They met up with some long-time friends at another venue that had always held fond memories for them when they had holidayed there. These people were quite shocked in the decline in Mac's health.

Whilst the few days were a cherished memory for Jane, it was interesting that Mac did not once, want to be rude to his wife. He was quite happy to have Jane by his side. Small mercies give the greatest of pleasures.

Jane's daughter, Joanne, had requested a transfer with the education system back to the Sunny Coast, to be close to her mum. She had submitted that for medical reasons it would be appropriate to be close to Mac.

Her and hubby had bought a lovely home not far from Caloundra. She envisaged that Jane and Mac would move in there one day soon because it had a granny shack on the property. It was self-contained and would be suitable. That way they would be close when Mac needed extra help to get through the challenging times.

She knew her mum was close to falling apart and not being able to continue with care for Mac, if she was not to get some sort of break.

Christmas was almost upon them again. Jane's daughter, Tia, who lived in Brisbane wanted her mum and Mac to come down to celebrate. Jane declined. The reasons behind most unaccepted invitations were that Mac could not cope with people, noise, and unfamiliar places. Joanne decided on a family Christmas celebration, and it would be easy for Jane to drive over from their unit and stay for most of the day. Mac could still have a snooze if he got restless.

That Christmas Day proved to be a bigger disappointment than the holiday away for a few days. Mac was unsociable and it was easier for Jane to return home well before the anticipated time. Still there were some lovely photos for memories.

The daughter in Brisbane asked could she come up to stay for a few days over the first days of the new year, since the Christmas celebration had not been put into practice.

Jane thought it a reasonable request, but all the while she feared Mac would be unsociable and could present a problem. He did. He once more became agitated with the extra people's noise. Unfamiliar faces each day and activity in the usually quiet unit. It was never that he didn't love them. It was only the fact that he forgot who they were and how they came to be in his house.

Once more Joanne approached Jane and asked her mum would she consider moving from the unit at the beach into the granny shack. Jane did not have to give this a lot of thought; she knew the many times that Mac had proven that he was demanding with everyday needs were becoming more regular and the prospect of full-time care was looming, quickly.

Jane had responded that she felt it would be her that would be moving into the granny shack once Mac was in care, but in that moment, she realised that she knew little about the procedures pertaining to this change.

Together they made the necessary phone calls to many places, and whilst Mac was at respite, they would visit some of the homes looking to see if all the needs of Mac would be catered for. One morning when they were sitting having coffee downtown, Jane got a call from Blue Care Caloundra. They were offering a place for Mac. Permanent stay. This was one of the places that Mac's doctor had highlighted as having adequate dementia care.

Jane could not believe it. She did not want to believe it. Her daughter took the call as Jane was suddenly pushed into acceptance of what life had become and what the future was offering for them all. Joanne listened and learned all of what had to be done legally. It had to be done within twenty-four hours.

Jane sat looking at Mac as he struggled with his cup of coffee. Mac was going away. Into care. Jane could only sit and recall how quickly the decline had taken shape. Some three years previous Jane had been advised to get 'the power of attorney' into play. At that time, Mac had barely managed to write his name. Jane knew right at this stage; Mac would not know how to even begin to write anything. He still knew his name but within another day, he would not remember his new address.

Mac went into care the day after Valentine's Day 2017. Jane would never forget the significance of that day.

The day before he went in, Joanne's family, Betty, Jim and Jan, had all come for a Valentine's celebration after the kids finished school. Soft drink and cakes and chocolate. Mac was pleased to see the grandkids. They had not been told what was happening the next day. Neither had Mac. He was oblivious to everything.

That night was the hardest night that Jane had lived in the unit. She slept little. Preferring to sit up and read and watch her darling man, slumber on beside her. Life would never be the same, she knew that, but what she didn't know was that the life ahead of her and Mac, would be full of more severe dementia displays and the love that they shared for one another would be filled with agonising moments and further sad and lonely times.

Individuals with severe dementia will not hold conversations. They may utter a few words and phrases especially if it is about something of interest for them. Rarely will they relate to their current environment. Most patients will need assistance with all their daily living activities. They will need help with bathing, dressing and if they were left alone would not be able to complete the task of getting a meal for themselves.

Often the patient will become argumentative with possessions. Believing everything to be only for them. When Jane had read many stories about dementia patients, an interesting one had been on possessions.

Often the patient will become aggressive, believing that they own everything. Like naughty children, they do not share.

The last visit for Jane to Mac's lovely doctor, before Mac had gone into care, he had described the dementia stage in a way that made Jane sit up and take notice. He described the patient as writing the script. That patient was in charge. He/ she was the main star. It was their drama they were performing. The carer must learn the lines. Those lines could change with the drop of a hat. No day would be the same. Same people, different script. Learn to be an actress/ actor and get into the role of the playmaker.

Jane wondered what Mac would write in his head for his next act. Little did she know it was nearly the final act.

Chapter 12 - The Big Blue Room Behind That Locked Door

If ever a moment was etched into Jane's mind, it was the day that Mac went into permanent care. Blue Care Caloundra was a busy place. A place for people who were ageing gracefully and some, not so easily. There was a section that was a retirement facility and another for someone who needed full time care. Then there was the wing where Alzheimer patients lived. Jane looked upon it as the blue room behind the locked door.

It was locked so that the in-patients could not get out and wander. Within that space behind the solid door, lived ten and sometimes, twelve patients. Some women, some men. Varying stages of the debilitating disease. The infirm, some frail. Some more lively than others. Some having lived there for years whist dementia eroded their normal life.

Mac had no idea what was happening that morning. Neither did Jane. She had rung his daughter, Marie, and she had come up from Byron Bay to see her dad. To say hello. To say good-bye.

Jane had packed his bag of odds and ends. Following a given list as a guideline, she had not had a big bag. It was filled to the brim, over-flowing with Mac's favourite shorts and shirts. His toiletries. Shoes for comfort as well as slippers. She'd not really wanted to dwell on packing that bag.

Whilst Jane had been getting Mac to the home, Joanne's husband had delivered Mac's favourite recliner chair to be placed in his room along with a chest of drawers, a portable tv and a portable cd player with his favourite CDs. Joanne had brought with her, some interesting photos and paintings to be hung on the walls. One's that Mac would recognise. They had bought a special doona cover and special pillowcase, for his bed, and all to make the room, homely, something he'd get to know as his.

Jane had to attend to paperwork relating to Mac's in-care. Marie and Joanne had sat with Mac in the blue room having a coffee and morning tea. He'd been quiet whilst he looked around him. Saying very little, but mostly asking where he was at. He did keep asking why he was there? He did keep saying that he wanted to go home and find Jane!

The girls talked to him quietly and assured him it was a respite facility like the one he had been attending twice a week. This one, that they were sitting in, was a little different but that is all they had offered in way of explanation at that time. Both were feeling quite awful. Understandably!

Once Jane had finished the meeting with the head clinical sister, and other staff that would be in attendance to Mac's needs, where she had discussed Mac's daily routine, his likes, his dislikes, she was free to join all of them behind the locked door. Mac got up as though to leave once he recognised Jane.

She made a point of taking him for a walk down the hallway to find his room. Joanne had put Mac's clothes away and his chair was in place. Mac went straight to it and sat in it. He put his head back not saying a word.

They talked amongst themselves. Quietly, while Mac dozed. They realised to get out of there without Mac was going to be a huge problem. They were saved from the delicate situation. One of the nurses came to get Mac and suggested she had something of interest to show him with some of the other people living there. He was reluctant but he went anyway. It was their cue to leave.

"Come back anytime, no matter what," they had all been told.

One of the senior aged care personnel in charge, had prompted them to share as much as possible about Mac, to make their chore of looking after him, that little bit easier. She had been made aware of some of his outbursts.

She talked quietly about all the patients behind that door. They were all individuals, but they all had grief at different times of the day and expressed it in varying ways. Time would tell as to how Mac would settle in; they did not expect it to be a breeze; they knew that dementia patients do whatever the moment prompts them to do.

It had been easy to talk with the senior carer person, Joyce was her name. Jane was to become very close to this carer. She had been working in the facility for many years. She had seen people come and go. Nothing surprised her anymore. She encouraged Jane to come back and visit when she was ready to.

If she felt she could not cope, then Jane should stay away. They would all understand. Never should Jane feel obliged that she had to be by Mac's side, twenty-four seven. Jane needed a break, as well.

Jane shared with that carer, that the afternoons were her hardest. Mac turned into a monster when the sun went down. She'd prefer to come and see him of a morning, but she was worried how once she was in there, her escape into the real world would become a problem for Mac and her. She was assured there were ways with words and ways of dealing with 'out-of-the-norm' behaviour.

Once inside the blue room, there was a locked kitchenette. All meals were prepared down the other end of the building in a bigger kitchen and brought up to the dementia wing.

However, this kitchenette was equipped with crockery and cutlery, glasses and cups, cereals for breakfasts and loads of preserves as well as cordials, tea and coffee, for all. Electric appliances, microwave, fridge, a double sink, and a huge bench where the meals were assembled for the in-patients.

There were four round tables with comfortable chairs, placed around in an open plan area. Recliner chairs were pushed into another spacious area. A huge tv mounted on one wall. There was a piano. A radio/cd player and bookshelves with books. There was a wall unit which housed puzzles and games and jigsaws and every imaginable creative piece for the patient's pleasure.

In one corner of the entry room once inside, there were two prams complete with dolls and a chest of drawers that housed some of the best doll's clothes ever made for any size doll. Jane thought that odd, but she was to learn before too long, how those prams and dolls were the most cherished possession of a couple of the ladies who lived in there.

The eating area was painted brightly, and the furniture was comfortable. In that area there was also a medical supply room that always remained locked. Further to the right there was long enclosed desk where rotating staff sat and did paperwork, answered phones and generally observed the in-patients.

Past this area down one hallway, there was a toilet and huge bathroom. Adequate bedrooms on each side.

Back around past the piano and tv watching area, double sliding doors led out to a paved area with outside tables and chairs. Over Mac's stay this area was upgraded from that first rough and uneven pathways to beautiful gardens and seating areas were put in place for everyone to enjoy.

Back inside again, past the piano another hallway went to the right. Toilets and bathrooms. A washroom for pans and personal hygiene utensils. A storeroom with bits and pieces of equipment such as wheelchairs and lifting machines Then six bedrooms, three either side of the hallway, Mac's room was down that hallway.

Time Zone

The big blue room,
And an always locked door
What lay ahead
What was in store
For me?
Never mind he had no friends
No timepiece to count down a day
We were all actors
This was his play.
Books lay open
On a table here and there
A piano sat waiting for cue
There was a garden outside, tended with care.
Recliner chairs, some red, some blue.
"What is this place?" he said to me,
"I've no time to sit and chat
I need to be home, but....
I can't remember where it's at!"
I assured him that the day was good
I watched a simple meal be served,
How was I supposed to say,
That a bed within had been reserved
And here he was to stay.
I contemplated life that day
For him as well as me
I was the one who shed the tears
As I turned and walked away.
I was the one, who lingered long
It was I who wished to stay.
I would have the broken heart as I kissed him on the cheek
I would hide my tears I'd wept, as I found it hard to speak,
"See you soon, my love, I'll be gone a little while

Rest, and have a nap
I'll be back before you know it,
I'm going searching for your cap."
Some days he knew me,
and I played his game,
especially when he forgot me,
when he gave me no real name.
His words became singular
No malice, no spite,
Each day was different,
Some jovial, some bright.
But I tucked away each memory
I held fast to the life that had been
For all that he did was so unprepared
So off hand, so unforeseen.

Chapter 13 - Life! Love! Loss!

It took Jane two days to get her head around not seeing Mac. She rang the home on both days to inquire his mood, his acceptance of his new place to live, and general well-being.

The staff were reserved in their judgement but offered that he was well and appeared to be settling. They did not push for her to make a commitment to coming in to see him.

It had been very quiet in the unit without Mac. Jane had gotten up early the next morning and went for a big walk to the beach. These walks would become a normal routine. Her time to reflect on the day before. She had a lot of thoughts to put into the right compartment of her mind.

More than once, Jane agonized over the fact that she had put him in the home. She felt lost. Jane could almost hear Mac's fear at being lost. He would be lost without her, that was a given.

The biggest hurdle that Jane had to jump over, was facing him once more on different terms.

Sure, he would be out of sorts and out of character, but would he, she wondered to herself. Had he travelled so far down the tunnel that a day was not twenty-four hours anymore. No definition of when to do the things he would have done at home with Jane.

Not that they had done things methodically either, but it had a routine that he would have been somewhat used to. Perhaps.

Only way to find that out was accept her lot in life and get on with the play that Mac had been performing for the last eight years.

She wished, not for the first time, she had a little crystal ball. Not to tell her everything, only a hint as to what to expect.

Jane had been happy in her own mind, with her decision to go into the home in the mornings not afternoons. Watch and learn the procedures. Get to know the staff. Observe the other inpatients. Learn some names.

Jane was not an out-going person. Shy and reserved, she often came across as not wanting to partake life's life with gusto. Jane would stand back in the queue and let many go before her. Going into the home was a challenge for her as much as Mac.

Learning the procedure into getting into the 'blue room' did not present too many problems. People were coming and going all the time. It was harder to get out. Though many often tried to do that.

Instantly inside the room she was approached in a menacing way by a woman shaking a fist at her.

"Get away from my baby. Don't you touch my baby! Get out, go on. Go away!"

What the hell! Jane stepped around the pram parked in the walkway into the open plan area. Once more the woman shrieked at her, 'GET AWAY FROM MY BABY'.

Jane stopped. Looked around for someone to ask "Hey, what's happening here?" but no one seemed perturbed. She peered into the pram. A doll lay snuggled in a lacy blanket. Jane looked up at the woman.

"Oh! she is so beautiful. What is her name? I bet I know, is it Rosy?" Jane asked.

This woman, who Jane thought looked every bit of seventy plus, did not commit to answering her, but she was no longer aggressive and was quite happy to pick up the doll and nurse it, leaving the pram still in the way.

Jane went to move it, then thought better of it. Another older woman came up to her.

"What's your name, luv? I like getting visitors. Are you visiting someone?" she asked all the while rubbing her hands together like she was anxious about something.

"My name's Jane, and I can't even guess what your name could be. You'll have to help me. Actually. Could you help me? Would you tell me some names of the people here. I don't know anyone."

She walked towards the chairs seated at the tables. She sat on one then pulled out another one beside her and turned to the lady that had spoken nicely to her,

"Come and sit beside me and tell me a story. Can you do that?"

Her name, Jane discovered was Ada. Ada had been at the home for two years and she was the one who played the piano. Not all the time. She had to be coaxed but she played brilliantly, apparently.

She pulled Jane close to her and suggested Jane did not speak to the lady with the doll. "She's mad, that one." She said with conviction all the while nodding her head and still rubbing her hands together.

Jane took a moment to have a look around the room. There was no sign of Mac. She'd get to him soon enough. Firstly, she had to get past the 'mad one'. Over at the next table there was another man sitting looking at a magazine. He did not appear that interested in it. He kept looking at Jane. Not in a bad sense, but it took another few minutes for Jane to find her voice and say 'hello'. He nodded but didn't speak. Kept on looking at her.

Over in front of the tv on the wall, there were a couple of ladies falling asleep in recliner chairs. There was a bit of noise coming from the kitchenette and Jane got up from the table and wandered over to the servery/counter and looked for someone to speak to.

One staff member was cleaning up the remnants of what Jane guessed had been morning tea. A trolley was packed with plates and cups and glasses. A young girl looked up and said, "Can I help you?"

"Good morning, I'm Jane, Mac's wife. I thought I'd come in today and see him. How's he been?"

"Gee, I can't answer that. I'm from down the other end, got to return this trolley to the kitchen down there. You'll find someone down the hallway, probably in the bathroom or toilet area. Or they could be outside. Go for a wander, I'm sure someone will speak with you."

Jane turned around and had a better look about. With that, one efficient looking carer came bustling out from down the hallway. She looked at Jane in an inquiring way. Once more Jane introduced herself.

"Mac's outside. In the garden. He's been helping sweep. You can go out there if you want to. There are tables and chairs to sit at. A nursing assistant like me will be out there. Or one of the registered nurses will be down in the bathroom area. Want to see someone?"

"No. Not particularly only wanted to see how he has settled. It's all a bit new for me. Not sure of the procedures expected."

"Jane, nothing is expected of you. You can come and go as you please. Take your time getting to know us all. I expect at first, it'll be hard. You'll get to know who to steer clear of!" she laughed.

"Yep, already encountered the woman with the doll, she was a bit full on! And I've met Ada."

"Ada's a darling. She is quiet most days, but if she takes to you, you could be lucky and get her to play the piano. Crazy lady with the baby, is Doris. She's been here for three years. Thinks she owns the place. She's mostly harmless. Gets upset about her baby, but it passes as quickly as it comes about."

"Well, I discovered that straight up. She hums to herself all the time," Jane offered.

"Yes, Doris used to be a chorister. Beautiful voice, apparently. Now she only hums. No family to speak of. A distant son who lives in NZ, so she gets no visitors."

The assistant carer who was chatting to Jane went on to relate some of the aspects of the other patients that Jane could see from where she was standing. Not on a personal level. Mainly for Jane's benefit for future reference. With that a man came shuffling down the hallway. He only had boxer shorts on. He looked about eighty.

"Mr. Wright. Go and put some clothes on please. It's nearly lunch time and you can't come to the table dressed like that! Come on, I'll help you find a shirt, shall I?" the woman turned back to Jane and extended a hand to her.

"I'm Tina. Nice to meet you. Go and see if you can find Mac. I'd better look after this man or Ada will get cranky with him. She hates him wandering around with no clothes on."

Jane found Mac sitting outside in the garden area. He looked up at her. Recognition not instant, then a dawning light and a smile lit up his face. Jane kissed him on his cheek. He patted the seat beside him, and she sat down. It took all her will not to start tearing up.

"How are you, Mac? Been sweeping I see. It's windy today, I think you'll have a big job to sweep them all."

He didn't comment, kept looking at her but she recognised the tune he tried to start whistling. It had been a favourite of his. He did not whistle like he once did. Yet, Jane knew and believed he knew who Jane was in that precious moment.

The senior carer, Joyce, who had been out there with Mac and two other people, was the lady that had been so helpful on the first day of entry. She came up and sat beside Jane.

"Hello, it's lovely to see you again. He's been calling for you all morning. And all yesterday. It's nice to see you here. Mac's been a bit naughty but nothing that we can't look after. He likes to pace up and down the hallway, calling out your name."

Jane picked up Mac's hand and held it between hers. He winked at her. Her heart lost its beat. She did not have to speak. She only wanted him to know that she cared for him.

"Stay for lunch with him. You can sit beside him. Chat with him. If you ever want to have a meal here with him anytime, that can be arranged. The kitchen is always ready to please. Before you leave today call and see me out in the main area, and we can talk over some things."

With that she got up and went inside. Jane continued to sit with Mac looking at the other man who was sitting with his wife not far from them. The wife was propped up in a recliner bed. He acknowledged Jane's presence but did not speak. The woman was not talking, and she appeared to be asleep.

Jane let her eyes wander around the outside area. It was certainly in need of repair. She had been told that a maintenance project was in the pipeline and looking at the uneven pathways, Jane guessed it would not be before time.

Still, it was quiet sitting there. Big gum trees lined the fence further away, and Jane realised that was where all the leaves were coming from. She could hear the chatter of birds and instantly knew why Mac would find it easier to sit outside rather than inside.

For the first time in many years, Jane found it hard to find the right words to say to him. She recognised the fact that if she talked about the place as though it was new to him, it may trigger him to not want to stay.

It was also hard to ask him what he had been doing. He would not remember. She must study this new script of his, very closely, for she knew she was one who would have to initiate conversation. Not Mac.

Jane sat back and watched a couple of ladies come outside. They were pushing walkers. They could not walk too far because the path was uneven, so they ventured down a little way, turned and came back. They stood in front of Jane.

One spoke, "You with him? He's loud. Always yelling."

Now Jane did wonder how to reply to that question. She thought she'd distract the lady by saying,

"I love your pretty dress. Someone must think you are special because the dress suits you."

The lady looked down at her dress. Nothing excited her about the statement Jane made. She opened the front part of the walker and Jane was privy to what was stored inside. A hankie and a purse, and a bag of chocolates. The lady opened the bag of chocolates and gave one to Mac. He looked at her for a beat then slowly opened the chocolate.

"Thank you!" said Jane. "Mac loves chocolates. Do you have a name I can call you?"

"I love chocolates too," replied the woman, but did not offer a name.

Jane realised more than ever how hard it must be to communicate with some people with dementia. They live in their own world, and sometimes that world is filled with silence.

The lady that was following the one with the chocolates spoke up, "Her name's Hettie and I'm Jenny. We go everywhere together. We've been playing quoits with other people. You could bring Mac down sometime, if he wants to come with us."

"Oh! that would be lovely, how do you get to this place?" Jane asked.

The woman was vague and waved her hand around to indicate somewhere. By this time Hettie was impatient with talk and pushed Jenny out of the way and made to go back inside. Jenny merely stepped aside and followed her.

Right in that minute Jane knew she had a million questions for staff to answer. In her mind she called these ladies Heckle and Jeckle. Not disrespectfully to their face. They accepted each other without preamble; they were good company for each other, but Hettie was the pushy one.

Lunchtime was as interesting as reading a good book. Jane was engrossed with everything. So much happening. Slowly people wandered to the table which had been set by a staff member. Place mats down and a plastic cup of cordial placed in front of it. Some men and women were helped by staff.

Ada smiled as she sat next to Mac. Jane was still standing behind Mac, watching. Staff brough a frail looking lady to the table. Her name was Mary. Nearly 100 years old. Holy cow! She been here in the home for years. She was not that demented but had flashes and this was home to her. A comfort zone with aid.

Mr Wright who had clothed himself, or with help, sat at the lunch table beside Hettie and Jenny. Another woman Helen sat to make up the four. Doris sat by herself until another woman came from up the hallway.

Jane had been told that staff discouraged patients spending hours in one's room. She was to learn that another woman, Jeanie, was there on a respite temporary stay. Her and the husband lived out west near Cunnamulla. She had only recently been diagnosed with dementia and it was a trial to see if she would settle in the secluded area, such as this dementia wing. She had become a wanderer and for her safe keeping, hubby had looked at the possibility of her becoming a permanent, as he could not look after her.

Staff encouraged the open area or outside, as a resting spot, for most hours of the day, unless they were doing activities that were supervised. Yet, there were a couple of ladies that obviously spent a lot of time on their beds. Doing what? Sleeping perhaps or watching tv.

The woman who was in the recliner bed, and who Jane had seen outside with her husband, was pushed into the eating area not far from the rest of the patients. Her husband proceeded to feed her though Jane noted it was not a full meal. Merely custard and jelly in a bowl.

Mac loved his meal. He'd always had a good appetite and it was obvious that moving into the home had not diminished his liking for it.

One of the staff sat beside Mary and fed her, she looked up at Jane and said, "Pull up a chair. Make yourself a coffee if you wish or get a cool drink."

Jane found a spare chair, but her mind was racing with all the different activity. She watched one husband get another drink for his wife, but the lady was not interested in food. Hettie and Jenny pushed their food around their plates. Particularly Hettie. She was "rail" thin. Obviously lived on chocolates.

Jane voiced a quiet question to the staff member who sat feeding Mary at the table.

"Where do they play quoits, Jenny was mentioning that her and Hettie had been playing this morning."

"Oh, that would be down the other end of this building. The people there are aged but not needing help, like the ones in here, so they have a lot more activities happening. We always ask who wants to go down there on any day, but usually they decline."

She went on to say that Mac would have been asked but he probably said no, indicating that he's not yet familiar with everyone. She suggested to Jane to go down there and look for a notice board that showed the weekly events.

"I certainly shall look for that because it might help Mac. There is so much to get my head around with everyone and everything."

"The other thing I was going to tell you was that there are volunteers who take the inpatients for a walk around the perimeter of this whole concern. It's a good walk."

"Would I be able to take Mac around by myself?" Jane asked.

"Of course. I can't see a problem with that. Ask one of the registered nurses if you can start doing that. I noticed Mac likes being outside."

"Yes, he does. We have always walked a lot of the times before he came in here. It might be good for him, tire him out!"

Jane remembered when they had first come to live in Caloundra. Their unit was not far from King's Beach and Mac had loved the walk. At that stage to get around to the next beach, Bullcock Beach, one had to walk some beach then scramble over rocks, not accessible when the tide was incoming, but over the years a wonderful boardwalk had been put in place and it offered great ocean views as far away as Moreton Island.

The vista to the west as one walked took in the imposing and impressive Glasshouse Mountains. The boardwalk finished on the edge of what is known as Happy Valley. A shady and cool area set aside for holiday makers, day visitors to the beach and perfect for celebrations of any kind. BBQ facilities and a playground for children.

Jane sat wistful for one moment remembering walks with Mac.

After lunch it was rest time. Usually, a movie was selected on the big TV or residents could sit in one of the recliner chairs and listen to quiet music playing. Jane wondered what Mac would do.

He got up from the table and headed towards the toilet area. She did not want to leave without saying good-bye, but instinct told her to go and have a talk outside with the head nurse. She noted he was unattended walking towards the toilet area. He was hesitant, walking very slowly, yet he did not seem lost. Jane thought about her once vibrant Mac.

She chastised herself. *'Stop it!'*

Chapter 14 - Progression...Regression

When Mac had gone into the home, Jane had a few last weeks at the unit that had been their home for fifteen years or more. Joanne and her family had urged Jane into moving into the Granny Shack adjoining her daughter's place.

This was a big move. It was nostalgic and a huge number of memories were left behind in the unit. Jane realised the move had to be for the right reasons, mainly because she would not be able to afford the rent at the unit, as well as pay for Mac's home accommodation. She settled easily, albeit differently.

The new living arrangement took place a week before Easter. It was decided that they would bring Mac out from the home for the morning and lunch on Easter Sunday to Joanne's place. Jane knew that it was an accepted practice at the home for families to offer outings and then return the inpatient later in the day.

Whilst Mac had been happy to sit and watch Joanne and family members come and go, he dozed in a comfortable chair. He had a beautiful meal and generally fit the day. The upheaval came when they took him back to the home.

Never had Jane envisaged that a problem would, could arise. She naively presumed that Mac would accept his return to his new abode. Wrong! He yelled and carried on, not wanting to go inside and when he was eventually coaxed into sitting at the table ready for dinner with a cool drink and a sweet biscuit, Jane and Joanne left to go back home.

Mac spent a very distressed night and staff had not been able to subdue him for many hours and then only after he had been administered a mild sedative. The next day when speaking with one of the staff members, Jane was quietly advised that sometimes a trip away can be most stressful for the patient and, as well, staff then have a herculean job getting them back under control.

She was not forced into believing that to partake of this practice would cause problems and it was never suggested, but Jane got the underlying message.

Jane and her daughter never took Mac out of the home again. Someone always visited him at his place.

Jane received a phone call a couple of days after this incident saying that Mac had had a fall. He'd been outside and stumbled on the uneven path. He had not injured himself to any great degree, that is, there were no broken bones, but he had gashed his shin severely and his doctor had been called in for an examination.

Jane did not want to make waves, as in, voice her opinion too harshly, but she knew Mac had always held her hand whilst walking everywhere. Not so much in the unit, daily walks namely.

She had noticed that Mac often shuffled unattended to the toilet.

When she had offered to take his hand, on more than one instance, he had shaken it away and he had preferred to walk unaided.

Jane understood some patients will not accept help as their crawl through the tunnel becomes evident. They still feel themselves to be invincible. Now that this accident had happened, Jane wanted answers as to why Mac had been left to stumble on that uneven path.

Her questions were answered thus, 'Mac had been calling and calling for Jane. He had become agitated and after a few up and down the hallway rants, had wandered outside probably before staff realised, he had gone, or maybe they thought outside would calm him down. They never envisaged he would have that fall. He'd been quick and in his agitated state had obviously not really looked where he was going.'

Did Jane want to accept this statement? Part of her did, because she realised, he had been very unaccepting of his living arrangements, since the outing at Easter. He had not calmed down from his anguished state. If anything, he had been even more distressed, more often.

She knew the patients did not have a one-on-one attendant, and it would be virtually impossible to watch each one, every given moment. And, given that Mac had been having one of his regular yelling sessions, she could see in her mind and believe, what had happened.

When Jane spoke with the head nurse and listened to the sorry tale, she had stressed that he needed help in walking any distances. He simply could not move his legs that easily anymore.

Staff suggested that a walker may help. Jane sat confused. Had they not picked up that Mac's sense of direction was askew?

Now Jane was, by no means a medical person who had a certificate, but she was aware after living with, and guiding him for the last few years, that Mac would not be able to push a walker, let alone guide it correctly. His spatial awareness was shot.

Jane made a statement; Mac could not walk unattended. Could staff please help here and recognise that this would have to be addressed. Simple as that.

Jane also knew in her heart that day that she would have to come into the home every day, from that day on, before morning tea and stay until after lunch when Mac would most likely have a little nap. This would give her some peace of mind. It would also help staff who were over-stretched in their daily chores.

She again stated that she preferred to not be in the home in the afternoon, not wanting to deal with his anguished requests for *'where is my wife? Find my wife, please!'*

After the accident to the leg, Mac was restricted in his wandering. When Jane came into the home, Mac was usually sitting in a recliner chair. With his head back listening to the music playing nearby.

Jane guessed he must be hurting more than he could tell anyone, for if she touched around the affected area, Mac grimaced and yelled out. Jane spoke to the head nurse and requested that the doctor be called again to have a further examination.

The area had become infected, and Mac was given a course of antibiotics. It took another week, and with constant supervision and medication, he slowly improved and was almost back to his cheerful self.

Jane discovered another aspect of the severe dementia had crept in whilst Mac had been sitting sedentary. His ability to move even to the toilet when necessary had reached the level that Mac was now wearing incontinence pads.

Up until his entry into the home, he had had no trouble with urination on time. Jane had always known that this aspect was going to be a confrontation for them both, so, Jane was saved the argument that would have ensued. He simply had to wear them in his new abode and as much as he would have bucked the system, all jocks were taken away, and he had no other choice.

The sad part was that Mac had not recognised that he wore the pad and not jocks. If he had the urge to urinate, he would often voice the need to go to the toilet but often did not make it in time.

Jane hated having to tell him that it was ok and that he wore a pad. She doubted he understood.

Time was not an issue for Jane. She had no reason not to come into the home. Sure, she had little free time to herself, not of a morning anyway. It was of little consequence, because she had chosen that Mac needed her for his composure and because her being with him, did free up time for staff to attend to some other person's needs. It gave her small peace of mind.

Once his leg had improved and he was once more able to walk with some aid, Jane and Mac started their daily ritual of walking after morning tea and heading out and about within the grounds.

Towards the end of the walk, they would find a seat outside in the shady area and sit it out till time to go inside for lunch.

She knew the fresh air and exercise to be good for him. They talked little but Jane kept up the usual dialogue about special items of interest that they may encounter on the way.

The walks were not strenuous, and their excursions were only ever for companionship and peace of mind for Jane. The walk was enough to tire Mac. Usually ensuring a good lunch and a well-earned nap, afterwards.

Mac had been asked to participate in quoits, down in the other aged care area, several times, but after a couple of throws that went askew, he'd not been happy with this arrangement. That was when Jane decided they would do a daily walk together. She did this at the same time when other activities were in progress for other patients.

On a bus trip one day, once again, Mac had gotten sick. It was sad, Jane realised, because Mac had loved being driven everywhere, sightseeing, but something was amiss there, and it was easier to say that those trips were not to be for him anymore.

From time to time there were a couple of entertainers that came into the dementia wing and performed with guitar. Their revue included all old songs that suited the patients. On St. Patrick's Day they dressed in green, and the Irish songs were the best medicine for all. They sometimes played the piano and whilst they dressed up in their best attire, the audience were all decked out in their colourful clothes to suit the mood.

The tables were covered with pretty tablecloths and there were chocolates and cakes for all at morning teatime. Mac loved these sessions. He tapped his feet to the music.

He no longer sang, as such; he had forgotten most of the words, and it brought tears to Jane's eyes, but he remained happy throughout the concerts.

By the time five months had elapsed into Mac's stay, Jane was no newcomer to the procedures of the dementia wing. She knew every little moment that was happening in the mornings.

She did not have, however, knowledge of what went on once sundown closed the day. Jane always arrived early to make sure the tables were set for morning tea. She helped make the cordial or prepared the cups and saucers for the hot cuppa.

Jane helped in the kitchen clearing up after a meal and only if Mac allowed her that time. She could always see him. Jane talked to him as she helped clear the tables and he was happy to sit and wait for her to come back and sit with him.

Mac was always showered early before Jane arrived at the home. The beautiful staff that she had to thank for some of her own sanity, were two ladies called Marnie and Jo. They worked tirelessly with Mac.

They never once stopped showing Jane what to do, how to do, or even attempt to do something to help Mac. They never thought that Jane interfered. Believing that her input was a help. They shared stories of Mac's naughty behaviour, and they forever helped her escape when it came time for her to leave the room.

Up until that stage these ladies had been shaving Mac when he had a shower. Jane commented that she could help and do that herself, because one day Mac was complaining about whiskers on his face. His hair needed clipping and she found it easier to cut his fingernails rather than let someone else do that chore.

He never seemed angry with Jane's care and let her perform all the little tasks that was needed to make him feel special. He sat docile, never offering a word. Sometimes Jane asked if he felt ok and he always responded with a wink and a smile.

Whilst there had been progression with Mac's ability to adapt to his new surroundings, his regression into the dementia world was more noticeable. He needed constant help each day. His ability to communicate effectively was the biggest hurdle in his world. It was obvious when he listened to the music that played near his recliner chair that some songs hit a button in his foggy head, and he would start tapping his foot to the tune.

When a couple of patients who Jane had become friendly with, died, Jane had to adjust her way of thinking as well. Finality was not a word that Jane used in her speech.

At the back of her mind, she knew she would not have her Mac one day, but to dwell in that space would have left her not wanting to come into the home at all to see her man.

She had visited Mac's doctor and had a wonderful consoling talk with him. He was not God, nor did he have a crystal ball, but he had been truthful in believing at that stage, that Mac had perhaps little more than a year of his life left to endure. He further told her that it would be filled with further angst and declining health conditions.

His Parkinson's had not reached its brutal peak, but it certainly had hindered his movements. Mac struggled with getting to the toilet unaided in every aspect. Jane learned what to do and did it diligently without a backward glance.

Staff cajoled her and advised that they were quite capable of looking after his every need, but Jane felt easier in herself, if Mac accepted her way of looking after him, whilst she was in his presence.

He started to struggle with his knife and fork at meals, that Jane was present for, and it became easy for her to feed him without too much ado, or prompt him into helping himself. Jane had been determined that he would never be fed some of the minced up and blended nutrients that other patients were fed.

She believed, that whilst he could still swallow, Jane wanted him to have something of substance. He was able to polish off corn flakes for breakfast without making too much of a mess and sometimes he liked his scrambles eggs.

Mac had his favourite meals. He always cleaned up all his desert. If he had a good lunch, then Jane was not worried if he had very little later in the day. She knew it frustrated Mac if soup was served because he simply could not handle a spoon to mouth without mess.

Soup was often served for supper, so Jane suggested if soup had to be served, then in a sipper cup would be far better to drink from.

With the doctor's words echoing in Jane's head, she knew that with the slow eating habits creeping in, it was an obvious sign of cognitive decline.

Mac was not aware of new people, coming and going, so it was no loss to him. He lived in his own little world. He called for Jane every day. Constantly.

Jane had sat one day and asked how the staff who became attached to patients and then they died, got on with everyday care and not let it affect them. They always responded that whilst they had favourites it did not pay to become attached over and above their duty.

Mac's eyesight had become weaker, and he had very little idea of knowing what some things were in the distance. He responded to people's voices and touch. He listened intently to conversations if someone sat with him and talked about this and that, but he very rarely replied or made a comment. His days were filled with monosyllables.

Chapter 15 - Make believe it never happened....

To that date at the home, Mac was fortunate to have several visitors. Jane's grand children who Mac would have proudly told anyone they were his as well, came whenever Jane asked could they spare the time.

Jane's oldest granddaughter was a regular. She visited with her little one.

She had filled many memorable moments with Mac when she had been much younger. Always visiting in school holidays and Mac had loved every minute with her.

All were aware of his decline. He always smiled but recognition was not present, and it made it hard for the younger ones to accept some visits.

His daughter, Marie, came when possible and whilst he was not always fully aware of who she was, he recognised her voice and he responded to her laughter and quick sense of keeping the moment light throughout the visit.

Jane's daughters Joanne and Tia were there as often as their family commitments allowed those visits. They struggled with Mac's daily visible decline. Acceptance was a word that Jane encouraged them to get their head around.

Whilst she was a constant visitor to Mac, she did not see the obvious that non-regular visitors noticed. She encouraged them to keep the visits light and often. Rather than lengthy and tedious.

Mac was having a birthday early December. Jane was making a huge cake, enough for all, and bringing chocolates and as many grandkids as could make it would be there. What fun! There were soft drinks and balloons and music. The best part of the whole day was the outside eating area.

Much work had been done in providing and improving a new, comfortable eating area outside. Surrounded by gardens and safe paths and beautiful plants and water features, it was the ambience of the place that always kept the patients quiet. They loved it. Staff were happy to provide many meals out there if the weather permitted.

The memorable photos taken that day would become a constant reminder of how the day had played out and how Mac had been so happy to oblige with good behaviour and a cheeky smile.

It did not pay for Jane to think back to the seventieth birthday party at the beach. What a difference that time had made, not only to Mac but to all the family. What had that time, dripping minute by minute, done to each one of them?

Jane enjoyed all her time with helping in an around the patients. Sometimes she helped with craft work or jig-saw puzzles, but most times she preferred to sit beside Mac after she had shaved him and made him comfortable.

He dozed in his chair often, no longer the daily walks to fill in and break up a lengthy morning.

One day a lovely lady paid a visit to staff and to some of the patients she had become friendly with when her husband had been in the dementia wing.

He had died before Mac had joined the group. This woman was like a breath of fresh air, and without being nosy and asking, Jane guessed her to be in her late seventies. Her husband had been a resident there for close on three years.

She stopped and spoke with Jane, saying she knew how often Jane came into the room and knew what Jane did to help and she also knew how the staff loved Jane being amongst them. They all had sung her praises.

Jane accepted the heartfelt words but demurred and said she was doing only what her heart told her to do.

It was something that she needed to do to make her not being able to cope with Mac at home with her. She missed their old home environment.

The woman went on to share a strange thing which stayed in Jane's mind for many days to come.

This woman had said to Jane, "You'll do your grieving in here, Jane, daily. You will live his life and not like any of it, but you'll accept it, and you will love him and miss the old him, even more, but when he's gone, you'll not grieve as much for the loss, for you have walked and grieved along the memory miles with him."

Jane did not understand, yet here the woman stood in front of her, with a smile on her face. She was not doom and gloom. She spoke with vitality, she looked fresh and alive, not worn out, and Jane would never have guessed that her husband had passed on only a year before this visit.

Speaking with her favourite nurses, Jane, asked about the woman. They had filled in the missing pieces as to how the woman fit the picture. Her husband had been very much like Mac, suffering Parkinson's, yelling and screaming for her constantly, never knowing her, though. It was only when she finally sat beside him, he'd eventually slip into a state of semi-recognition.

She'd done much the same as Jane for her husband. No one had asked her to do it, she did it because she wanted to. Yes, she too, had spent many a day in tears, like Jane. Not knowing what to say next, not believing she was making a difference, not accepting what life was throwing up at her. Plodding along that memory walk. One step at a time.

Jane didn't think she was grieving whilst she watched Mac daily. Not like she had grieved when her son had died. She'd never caught that curved ball. She fumbled her way through life, not accepting the loss, that was him.

Then one day, she realised how much Mac depended on her. She knew then, that if her son had become dependent on her with his serious brain tumour, and not died suddenly, she would have had a horrible decision to make as to which person she would have spent twenty-four hours minding. She would have been torn with guilt either way. Life and death are never easy. Yet sometimes there is a silver lining.

No longer was Jane worn out with giving of her constant care. She had been thrown a curved ball with Mac's dementia status, and so far, she had fumbled her way through hanging onto it. Yet, she had the good people at the home to be thankful for.

They were constantly giving back moments in which Jane could breathe compared to how she would have been drawing ragged breaths if she had maintained looking after her husband when he needed professional help.

Each day, Jane knew, there were unrepairable moments. He was sedated repeatedly for outbursts. Jane hated to hear about those times. It was unfair. Sometimes he would deliberately look at her and spit venom when she tried to tell him that she really was his Jane. He simply did not understand. She had to be content with the moments when he was happy for her to sit beside him.

Sometimes she cried for those moments when it had all been rosy. Yes, she realised, what the woman said, was true, she was doing her grieving whilst he was alive.

Each day was an act. Mac wrote his own script. Most scenes were the same, with the same actors and actresses. If one is to believe that someone cannot know the person they have loved and lived with for twenty odd years, then it is only through true grit and determination that one does the daily ritual of putting up with that act.

It goes without saying, that life is not typecast, and one must be prepared to perform as good as the scriptwriter.

Chapter 16 - Once upon a Christmas time...

The week before Christmas the entertainers came back again, along with their jingle, jangle finery. They sang the morning away with hearty voices. A long table was set up with festive cheer.

There was fruity punch to drink and Christmas cake and shortbread as treats. Chocolates and lollies were strewn over the table. There were fine sandwiches with ham and chicken and ice cream and fruit for dessert. It really was a spectacular display put on by staff and the guests gave it their all.

Mac loved the Christmas Carols. His favourite The First Noel had him mumbling some lyrics. Jane was amazed. Never had he been able to utter as much as that morning. He held Jane's hand, and it took a huge effort on her part to not fall into a heap at his feet and sing her song of lament. Her favourite nurses spoke to her often, encouraging and giving her hugs. How she got through that morning was only God-given.

It was fortunate that special pre-Christmas morning had taken place, for Christmas day that year for Jane was not one to be written into the records as heart-warming. Her daughter Tia and her family had invited Jane down for Christmas Eve dinner and drinks. Staying the night and returning early the next morning to the home to spend the day with Mac. On the drive back up to coast, Jane's thoughts rested with other people out and about early, rushing to visit and be with loved ones.

A splendid roast meal was planned for lunch with all the trimmings at the home, and plum pudding with brandy custard and ice cream, for dessert. This alone was an added enticement to get the patients out of their rooms and sit at the decorated tables, well before mealtime.

Most had enjoyed ham and eggs with toast for a huge breakfast. Limited staff were available, but Jane was happy to know that Jo and Marnie, were rostered on for most of that day.

Jane had requested her meal as well, preferring to sit with Mac for that time and return home to Joanne and her family later in the afternoon and celebrate a late Christmas day meal with them.

It was not a good look to walk into that room that morning and notice that Mac was not sitting in his favourite chair. She looked for advice and was told that Mac had been performing most of the morning and had been sedated. He was in his room.

Jane went and sat beside his bed whilst he was sleeping off the effects of the drug. He was agitated in his sleep, so Jane had gone to the kitchen to make herself a coffee and speak with staff.

Mac had then woken and had started his antics once more, calling for Jane.

She was beside him in an instant, talking quietly to him, and trying to take his hand and help him shuffle down to the eating area. His recognition of her was absent and the more she spoke the more he became agitated.

Jane looked to staff for guidance, with the ever-present tears spilling down her cheeks. One of the most respected nurses of that home, pulled her aside. She suggested Jane leave. Go outside for a bit. Come back in an hour and see how he had improved or not come back. Her choice.

Jane went outside and rang Joanne. After relating the reception, she had received, she talked at length with her daughter, wondering what would be best to do from therein. Joanne and her family were at the beach, an early swim was something they often did since their arrival back on the coast. It was decided they would call into the home and see if the visit might be good for Mac.

The grandkids, were marvellous, still dressed in sandy beach attire, but very happy to be singing out loudly, magical Christmas wishes.

One must love the beauty of young children's eagerness.

They had Mac smiling and behaving within a few moments. They posed beside him for photos and shared chocolates whilst Jane took five minutes to regain her composure. How could one not be moved by such tenderness and special times?

Mac was happy to put his head back and doze after they left. Jane stayed on and shared quiet moments with him. He was not all that hungry. Any wonder, he must have eaten lots of chocolates.

Jane was happy to let some other person have her meal, and she asked could something be set aside for Mac for later in the day.

As she pushed the small amount of plum pudding around in the bowl with ice cream and fed what would have once brought him much delight, Jane knew it made little difference to her man. Any day, each day, is all the same to them.

Christmas that year was another turning point. This severe dementia stage can last upwards of two years. Motor skills, including the ability to walk, occur at this stage. Angry outbursts are more widespread, and the individual will feel extreme agitation.

Mac was stumbling more often. He had many falls. He had to have a sensor mat beside his bed installed so that staff knew when he was up and about. He did little except sit in his favourite chair.

One such fall resulted in a hospital visit which was traumatic. Jane and Joanne met the ambulance, that had collected Mac at the home, at the local hospital. He was in an extremely agitated state.

He was calling and yelling for someone to find his Jane. There was very little recognition when she arrived, but it was her voice that eventually stilled his behaviour.

Jane was embarrassed with his loud rantings and tried ever so hard to pacify him. Mac had to have an MRI because they feared he may have had an epileptic fit causing his fall as well as an x-ray to see if all his bones were intact. What a nightmare that proved to be. He was anxious and did not believe anyone was there to help him.

Medical staff were reluctant to administer a sedative until results of blood tests and MRI were to hand.

Jane hardly believed that she and Joanne could sit for hours on end until finally they were informed, they should return to their home, because Mac would be returned to the home early the next morning.

It was after midnight when Jane left the hospital. It was pointless to think that peaceful days would ensue. Mac developed a cold that went straight to his lungs. Doctor feared pneumonia, but with antibiotics he slowly regained some composure. However, it left Mac very weak.

It was now obvious that Mac needed more constant care. Jane started staying at the home well into the afternoon. She always helped with feeding him his meals and toileting. Then suddenly Mac lost the ability to swallow his tablets. Then, he refused them altogether.

Custard became an ever-reliable additive to ensure the tablets went down the hatch. Still, there were days when he refused to play the game, and he went without drugs and custard.

Chapter 17 - The Final Road

Sipper cups were a must. Custard pills, cold coffee. Scrambled eggs. No toast. Cool sandwiches. Diced chicken or corned beef with mashed potato. Ice cream and jelly by the bowl full.

Anything relatively easy to swallow without being disgustingly like gruel.

Jane fed it all to Mac and he diligently sat and pretended she was someone else. Not every day, there were moments where a wink broke her heart, and he found a chuckle deep within the recess of his mind.

One day Jane was about to shave Mac, she'd prepared him and was on the verge of starting, when he stopped her. He mumbled something and Jane felt he did not want her to shave him. She said as much. He nodded his head. Pushed her away. Then he looked at her. She asked was there someone better he'd prefer to do it. He nodded again and was getting agitated.

Jane picked up all the shaving needs. Collected the basin of water and took it away. She went and made a coffee and sat outside and made a call to her friend. Leaving Mac to sit by himself.

After she'd finished her coffee, and regained her composure, she went back in to stand in front of Mac. She leaned in close. Said, "Hello, want a shave today, Mac?"

He gave her the thumbs up.

Sleep patterns are often impacted. Sleeplessness at night will result in exhaustion during the day. Mac had taken to staying awake at night. Individuals do not realise any hour on any given day.

He had one of the night staff sit with him and this fellow was a blessing. He talked footy to Mac till the cows came home, and eventually Mac would sleep. He would sip cold coffee and sometimes the night nurse would dunk his favourite biscuits in the coffee and feed this to him.

These people were precious to Jane.

Jane always received a call at night from the home. The staff never failed in letting her know Mac's every move once the sun had gone down.

She still could not bring herself to be in there after dark. Mac was experiencing a lot of falls. His tremors from Parkinson's disease had impacted on the use of his legs and feet, and it was obvious he needed to be restrained somewhat in bed.

This was not something that Mac liked to happen. He always felt the need to wander when he chose to and sometimes staff were not on hand to monitor his every move.

Patients had come and gone in the home in the year that Mac had been a resident. Jane's favourite lady, Ada, had a severe fall and it eventually impacted on her mental health. She was mourned by all who knew her.

Two men had arrived after Mac had lost the capacity to communicate which was a shame, for they could have been company for him, had Mac felt the urge to be friendly.

One man who had a different strain of Alzheimer's to Mac, was a very loud individual with behavioural problems, and he disrupted the patients and staff at any given time. The family of this man found it difficult to settle into any nice routine with him.

The wife of the man reached out to Jane for help at times and it was Jane's friendship that made it easier for the woman to visit her husband.

Some staff did not respond to the patient or the family as one would like to happen. One can be forgiven for this attitude.

Not all days are clean sailing and the angst felt can be a sad indication of losing contact when it is vital that a bonding is necessary for keeping everyone happy.

When patients with Alzheimer's are living together, some good aspects emerge, like Hettie and Jenny. They trailed each other around twenty-four seven. They parked their walkers beside each other and sat together at all meals.

They did not talk, they linked.

Though it is usual for each to adopt his or her own everyday antics, sometimes that bonding helps the patient to live easier in the confines that Alzheimer's pushes the patient into.

It stands to reason, that if the individual with loud behavioural antics continues to abrase other patients, and upset a relatively quiet room, this then will be a trigger for other misbehaviours that will spread within a heartbeat.

Patients are quickly moved away from the volatile outbursts.

Not always does the dementia ship sail on tranquil waters. Jane learned over the year that there is not one person with Alzheimer's the same as the next. It is not like contracting Measles and Mumps.

Yes, it is a disease, but whilst symptoms are much the same, the individual is not. They each portray unique individual signs of having one of the most debilitating diseases of the brain.

With the slow and tedious decline of Mac's life, it had impacted on Jane's life as well. Once upon a fairy tale time she had enjoyed the company of her sister. They had enjoyed a comfortable and at most times, happy lifestyle.

Throughout years of milestones in growing up, having children, marriages, deaths and new companions, they had kept each other secured in happy moments.

When Mac had first started his funny behaviour, Jane had confided in her sister that she knew that all was not well with him. The idea that he had dementia was scoffed at as it was by a lot of other friends and relations.

Mac being forced into retirement, changed each other's lives.

No longer the coffee mornings that they would have shared thus far. No more movies at the cinema. Existing daily phone calls became a weekly event and then they too, dropped off because Mac had hated when Jane talked on the phone.

So, Jane had often brushed her sister off, not intentionally, sometimes, though, perhaps heartlessly. Jane would say that Mac needed her, and it was impossible to talk on the phone.

Depending on how the sister took that information, they could go weeks without a word. Sometimes she would call in with her hubby for a cuppa, but Mac had not been always comfortable with these arrangements, either. The situation fell apart and became extreme. Sadly, communication then became non-existent.

During the years that Mac was ailing, Jane's sister slipped into ill health. She had suffered Rheumatic Fever at an early age, and it had been an underlining and ongoing problem throughout her life; accelerating as she aged and causing many other aspects of heart disease.

Jane's sister was four years older. With no speaking, it was impossible for Jane to know that she was extremely ill until Jane's niece spoke to her, and advised Jane, that her mother was being admitted to palliative care and she was asking Jane, would she come and say, 'hello and goodbye'.

It had been three years since Jane had seen her sister. The world of the nearly dying is quietly and effectively controlled by comforting drugs to alleviate any pain.

The heartbreaking moment came when Jane touched her sister's cheek and spoke to her. Her sister acknowledged her, knew who she was, knew to say, 'I'm sorry' and they were words that stayed in Jane's heart forever and a day.

Her sister passed away that night. Jane attended the funeral the next week and delivered her emotional account of what life had been like with her only sister. She did not have time to grieve then or any other day because Jane returned to the home to look after and be with Mac.

He died three weeks later.

Chapter 18 - Bury the Memories

Jane's older friend, Betty, from the unit block where she had lived, had stayed loyal to both her and Mac. She came to the home when it was possible for her to visit Mac. Usually when Jane was there. Whether Mac recognised her, because his eyesight was continuing to fail, or whether he knew her by her voice, Mac always smiled when she said 'hello'.

Sometimes he'd look at her without speaking and put his head back and be comfortable with her chatting about trivial stuff. It didn't matter what she spoke of, he listened. He always had time for Betty.

One cold, wet and windy Sunday Jane had collected Betty from her unit, and they had arrived at the home as morning tea was being served. Over the previous week, Mac had been confined to a recliner bed. He thrashed at times when he felt the urge to get up.

His legs were obviously giving him 'hell'. Not that he said as much. He was in an agitated state, day and night. Sedatives were helping but not lasting the distance or giving him or anyone else, a quiet time.

He pushed aside angrily any offer of help to make him more comfortable. His anguished voice was an indication of his pain level. He had not been showered, only a daily sponge bath. He could not stand at all anymore. Mac had not eaten anything of significance for a couple of days.

He had been fed jelly and custard and ice cream and yoghurt. Sipping sustenance drinks and then not really enjoying any of what was offered. Jane had been with him for most of each day, witnessing the decline. Yet, that Sunday was a show of fear and pain. She felt and heard his upset state.

Mac eventually slept when a stronger pain killer and sedative had been administered. Jane went home with a heart still lingering beside her man. The friendly head nurse had advised her that to get some rest might be a good idea, for she felt that Jane would be needing some extra strength over the next few days.

The previous week had been a roller coaster ride of emotion. Jane did not know what truly was happening, but she feared that something horrible was about to take place. The phone call from the home that night suggested to Jane that she should come in early the next morning.

When Jane arrived on that Monday morning early, she was immediately shown into the office area where she had sat sixteen months previously and signed Mac into the home.

She was told that Mac would be going into palliative care and Jane needed to read all the legal requirements and sign her consent to further drugs, namely Morphine, being administered.

The doctor had been called through the night and his decision had been that Mac's state had declined enough for this next stage to be put in place.

Jane sat in stunned silence, not wanting to state the obvious.

Finally, when she found her voice she said, "How long do we have?"

"How long is a piece of string? Who knows!" came the reply.

They offered a day or two, maybe more. Mac had a strong heart; it was the rest of his body that would shut down before that final beat.

Jane walked slowly up to Mac's room. The curtains were drawn, and the room was stilled into a quiet ambience. He was asleep.

She reached up and kissed his cheek. He murmured something. What? Maybe he felt she was there. Jane always wore the same perfume. Had done so ever since he had been diagnosed with Alzheimer's. She'd been told to do that at some point. Jane knew he could determine her smell.

She opened the curtains to let in the light. Mac had hated the darkness way back, before he had come into the home. He'd become fearful once the sun went down. Pulling back the blinds and opening doors to let light in. He'd loved the mornings. He'd been better of a morning too. Easier to look after and communication was acceptable.

Jane went and made herself a coffee and set about making the phone calls to the immediate family and friends. That task was easier than she first anticipated. Resignation of the inevitable was creeping into her heart and Jane was responding sensibly.

Strangely, the hardest conversation, that Jane had, was with Mac's sister. She had not believed her brother could have gone downhill so fast, for she had been to visit him for Easter only a couple of months beforehand. With her own husband's illness, one knew that it was only a matter of time before the final breath would be taken. He had had cancer and his death whilst not predicted on the day, had been close to an approximated date.

With Alzheimer's there is very little recognition that the end is near, unless it is spurred on by a weakened heart, or as in Mac's case, Parkinson's, or another underlying condition that will cause the body to shut down before the brain.

Mac's daughter, Marie, decided to come up and asked to stay at Joanne's place. It would make the time easier if Joanne didn't mind and Tia had already decided to have time off and to do likewise. Jane talked quietly with everyone. Then she was exhausted.

Her favourite nurses came and sat and talked to her. They suggested she go home for a rest and come back later in the day.

That seemed like a good idea once Joanne spoke with her, stating she was coming into see Mac as well that afternoon. She had asked for the rest of the week off from her teaching duties.

Mac was awake when Joanne and Jane arrived later that afternoon. He'd been shaved and had been given a sponge bath and change of shirt and bedclothes.

Whilst he was not responding to their talk, he knew he had company, and he was in a happier state than what the day before had presented to them all. They talked amongst themselves. Laughing and keeping the talk cheerful. Mac dozed. The doctor had been and had kept a watchful eye on developments.

When Jane suggested that the grandkids should visit if they wanted to, the next day was set for a succession of visitors from Jane's family. All within a reasonable time of each other, and not for any great length of time.

The atmosphere was pleasant, and Mac had responded to the kid's chatter and had offered a slight acceptance of their presence.

To Jane, Mac looked hardly different over a twenty-four-to thirty-six-hour period. She didn't know what she was supposed to be looking out for. His colour had changed. It had that greyish tinge which made her shudder if she thought too long about it.

She said as much to the head nurse. Once more, the quiet response was, "we do not know!"

Then the next morning when Jane arrived with Marie, Tia and Joanne, it was obvious that Mac's breathing was laboured, and she could hear a rattle in his throat. Medication was administered to help with this. The Morphine levels were increased marginally, and whilst the visitors went outside for a break, the nurses sponged Mac once more and changed his clothes and bed sheets.

Staff suggested that if Jane wanted to shave Mac, then she could do so. It filled in time and the girls laughed and offered a varied conversation throughout the afternoon. Mac slept on, somewhat fitfully, regardless.

An air diffuser loaded with a gentle, pleasant-smelling oil, was brought into the room and it offered a soothing ambience. Jane played on the portable cd player all the favourite quiet music that Mac had liked each day when he had sat in his recliner. There was a gentle hush in the room. Jane decided to stay the night.

It was a long night for Jane. She read her book, and listened to the music, drifting off to sleep eventually sometime after midnight.

The hustle and bustle of the dementia wing took on a whole new meaning at night. Listening to the other patients moving through their day and night was a reflective moment for Jane.

Remembering how Mac often used to prowl for a time unsettled.

That night Mac was restless and agitated so it was after 2am in the morning when the Morphine levels were increased a little, and then Mac had slept easier.

The girls had preferred to return to Joanne's home, as Mac's sister was coming up from the Gold Coast the next day and they were eager to be there with her for the visit. His cousin who had been one of the three musketeers in Mac's childhood adventures was to bring her up and visit as well.

Jane helped with the early morning routine at breakfast the next morning at the home, making some tea and toast and then had decided she would go home for a few hours' sleep. She then returned to the home to be with the girls who had gone in earlier. There had been little change with Mac in her absence.

From the Sunday before to that Thursday when his sister arrived, Mac had said little. He might have offered what seemed like a chuckle with the grandkids. He'd not said a word to Jane.

He had smiled if Jane prompted him that one of his favourite songs were playing and he should listen, but he'd slipped out of the real world for most of the time. The minute his cousin came into the room and boomed in his distinctive voice.

"Hey, Mac, what you doing lying there, mate?".

Mac was awake and aware. He laughed out loud. It was a deep throated laugh. It brought a moment of disbelief to all in that room.

His sister could not stop her tears. She cried and cried standing in front of Mac, all the while rubbing his shoulder and caressing his cheek. Mac knew her. He did not open his eyes, but he knew her. He seemed to respond to her.

It was moving, painful and affected everyone standing there. Jane went outside and left them to their cherished last moments.

Not for the first time, and again in that instant, Jane felt and wished Mac had responded to her in that way. Was it so unfair for him to not say, 'hey' back to her when she said as much to him?

She nearly collided with the head nurse, as she was hell bent on getting outside into the day. The nurse hugged her to her.

"Breathe" she said. "He knows you are with him. Believe me, he knows!"

That piece of string was getting shorter. Jane knew Mac was dying before her eyes. The morphine levels were very high now. No longer a twitch or a shudder or a shuffle of the bedclothes. No more the open eye. The persistence of death creeps in when least expected.

The family had contributed to well worked out moments when Mac's time would be up. They'd used numbers and minutes and hours and while the time ticked on and Mac still lived, they came together as a wholesome happy family and detailed the finer points of how the funeral would be and where it would take place.

It was in no shape or form, morbid. It was hilarious. They laughed and cried, and the doctor came and met all the family. He laughed with them. Some of the nurses had told them to be quieter remembering where they were and that there were other residents, but the doctor brushed it aside.

The doctor offered a smile to Jane. He encouraged the girls to be happy for their dad, because the worst part of his life was nearly over.

Jane was exhausted as well. Her heart had been broken so many times throughout the eight years of the dementia journey. It had been laced back together when the remembered good times had given her peace and understanding.

Now it slowed, keeping pace with Mac. She stayed another night and day and when late on the Saturday night the nurses suggested she go home, that maybe Mac wanted her to go home, to not be there when he passed out of his troubled world, she relented with reluctance.

The phone call came the next morning at 3.30am.

'Mac was gone. Come in straight away if she liked to be with him.'

Marie and Tia had said their good-byes on the Friday and Saturday. Joanne returned to the home with Jane. Mac's body was still warm when they got there. There are no words left to say to further enhance or diminish the moment.

They were given as much time as they wished to linger. Jane's tears had dried. By the time they left the home, the sun was coming up.

They got a coffee and headed for the beach. Mac's favourite place. They walked his beach. They found a significant shell.

A shell Mac and Jane would have collected many, many times on their walks. Their thoughts were sad but not hampered with injustice or anger.

Mac passed away on Seventeenth day of June, the year 2018.

When Jane scattered his ashes out to sea she wrote:

A cauldron of angst, a wild wash of foam, where is your spirit, where shall you roam?

Hear my whisper, heal my lament, the wind shall carry the message I've sent.

Send forth your beam, show me you're there, give me a sign, a sign that you care.

Jane pondered on what Mac would have said had he been able to speak:

Where shall I wander, to where should I roam, is there a space, a place of my own?

No more the tremble on this unknown path, ahead is a rainbow. No fear, no more wrath.

Look to the heavens, watch for flashes of light, look for the beauty in star filled warm nights.

No more the sadness, no acts of despair, show me the feelings of loving laid bare.

Show me the road that winds on and on, filled with such happiness to build up and upon.

Grant me a mantle, lined with silver and gold, to wear with conviction, pleasure sewn in each fold.

Give me new strength, find a good way, to erase all the sadness, that's plagued me each day.

After Note

In 2022 statistics reveal that worldwide, around 55 million people have dementia.

Dementia has physical, psychological, social and economic impacts, not only for the person living with it, but also for the carer, families and society at large.

Dementia is a syndrome – usually of a chronic or progressive nature. It leads to deterioration in cognitive function. It affects memory, thinking, orientation, comprehension, calculating, learning capacity, language and judgement.

Some health organizations state there are seven stages of dementia but basically, there is the early stage where common symptoms, include forgetfulness, losing track of time, and becoming lost in once familiar places.

Middle stage suggests that remembering events and people's names will impact on family and close friends. Increasing difficulty with communication, and possible help with personal care. Behaviour changes will include wandering and repeated questioning.

Late stage includes total dependency and inactivity. Physical signs and symptoms become more obvious. Unaware of time and place, recognition of relatives and friends, increasing need for assisted self-care, difficulty walking and behaviour changes may escalate and include aggression.

There are many different forms of dementia. Alzheimer's disease is the most common. Other major forms include Lewy bodies (abnormal aggregates of protein that develop inside nerve cells) and degeneration of the frontal lobe of the brain. Dementia may develop after a stroke, harmful use of alcohol and repetitive physical injuries to the brain. The boundaries between different forms of dementia are indistinct and mixed forms often co-exist.

The principal goals of dementia care suggest early diagnosis, optimizing physical health, cognition, activity and well-being. Understanding and managing behaviour changes is paramount and finally seeking and securing information for long-term support for carers.

Source: *World Health Organization*

Printed in Dunstable, United Kingdom